FROM THE AUTHOR OF

LIVE A
Beautiful Life
with
LUPUS

LUPUS *Diary*

Track Your Life with Lupus—
Body, Mind, and Spirit

OLIVIA DAVENPORT

CABIN CREEK PUBLISHING
RENO, NV

Dedication

This book is dedicated to everyone living with the mystery that is Lupus. May our lives be as full and beautiful as we are....

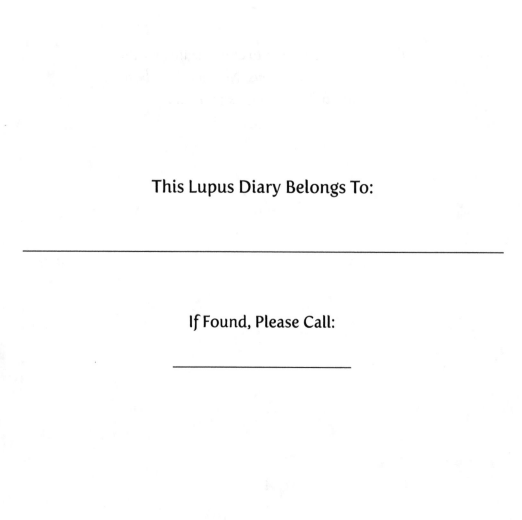

This Lupus Diary Belongs To:

_____

If Found, Please Call:

_____

Table of Contents

Introduction

No matter how you feel about diaries and journals, when you have an unpredictable auto-immune disease like Lupus, it's vitally important to keep track of how the disease impacts your life.

A May 2015 survey of Lupus doctors and their patients revealed a huge gap in how doctors perceive the impacts of the illness.* Doctors participating in the survey reported believing that their Lupus patients only experienced symptoms a few times per month; whereas, the Lupus patients participating in the survey reported experiencing symptoms *daily*.

That's shocking, right? How could there possibly be such a gap between our experience as patients and our doctor's perception? Either the doctors aren't listening, or we're not giving them enough information. Giving them the information about how Lupus affects us isn't easy unless we systematically keep track of our lives and symptoms. Keeping a diary is one way to do that.

If it's so important, why aren't all Lupus patients keeping a diary?

The problem with diaries has been that recording and tracking health isn't always easy or convenient to manage, especially when you're not feeling well. More specifically, keeping a health diary presents these typical problems:

- You're just not sure of what to write, or what's important enough to write.
- It's not easy enough to keep up with on a daily basis.
- It's too time-consuming.
- The typical blank-line format isn't helpful in organizing your information consistently.

A New Format to Help

This *Lupus Diary* format, which I originally created for myself, really helps overcome the problem of the blank page and has now become an easier way to help me remember all that happens to me between doctor appointments.

It's organized for tracking your health using prompts that guide you to make diary entries without worrying about what to write on a blank page, such as:

- Separate sections for body, mind, and spirit—to help you monitor your health holistically.
- Checklists for tracking your progress with the specific habits and rituals listed in the *Live a Beautiful Life with Lupus* framework—which serves as a reminder to take action to take care of yourself.

- A Meals section to monitor how your diet may be affecting your health.
- Inspiring quotes for each day, and more....

I hope you find this *Lupus Diary* as helpful as I have. Because I'm now able to express and explain myself by referring to the entries in the *Lupus Diary*, my doctor appointments have been more productive and less stressful. The added benefit is that I'm also more aware of how I'm feeling, how I react to foods, and what I can do for myself to feel better.

To get started, read and follow the instructions in the "How to Use" section on the next page. Then, as you complete each diary entry, enter the date for that entry in the "Table of Dates" on page 13 to give you a way to quickly reference a particular date when needed.

I invite you to visit my two websites:

- **Lupus Diary** online at *http://www.lupusdiary.com*. This is where, using the same format of this *Lupus Diary* book, I share the latest happenings in my life with Lupus—my triumphs, my setbacks, and everything in between. Although I keep my diary daily for myself, I only post a diary entry once a week on my website.

- **Live a Beautiful Life with Lupus** at *http://www.liveabeautifullifewithlupus.com*. This is where I provide inspiration and write about all that I'm learning about living and thriving with this autoimmune disease, as presented in my book of the same name.

Thank you, and all the best.

Olivia

* "Global Survey Finds Gap in Physicians' Understanding on Impact of Lupus on Patients' Lives." *News Medical*. News Medical: Health News and Information, 11 May 2015.

How To Use

Based on the framework of my book *Live a Beautiful Life with Lupus: Habits and Rituals for Thriving with an Autoimmune Disease*, the purpose of this *Lupus Diary* is to help you keep track of how you're feeling in a quick, easy-to-enter format that will be practical and helpful to you as you manage your life with Lupus.

Understanding that the idea of a diary, while important, isn't always realistic or easy when living with a chronic illness, the *Lupus Diary* is meant to make the most of your time and energy:

1. The *Lupus Diary* is designed to be filled out daily, if possible. If not, complete it as often as you can. It's best to complete it at the end of the day, when you can remember and reflect on your day.

2. The *Lupus Diary* is organized by the three dimensions of your being—body, mind, and spirit—to help you clearly distinguish what's happening with each part of your life.

3. In the "Body" section, write about your physical symptoms, vague or specific, as best you can, discussing if they are better or worse than the day before, unchanged, or new. Check off the habits and rituals of the *Live a Beautiful Life with Lupus* framework (see page 11) that you practiced to soothe your body.

4. In the "Mind" section, follow the prompts to express any cognitive symptoms, emotions, behavioral issues, or feelings that are affecting you that day—whether they are positive or negative. Check off the habits and rituals of the *Live a Beautiful Life with Lupus* framework (see page 11) that you practiced to strengthen your mind.

5. The "Spirit" section is where you record your pursuits at gaining inner peace and meaning beyond your physical and emotional symptoms. Follow the prompts, and check off the habits and rituals of the *Live a Beautiful Life with Lupus* framework (see page 11) that you practiced to nurture your spirit.

6. The "Meals" section is where you track what you're eating and how foods are affecting you. This is also where you record your daily intake of water.

7. In the "Notes and Reminders" section, write any thoughts about the day that you want to remember to discuss with your doctor during your next appointment.

8. The "Gratitude" section is where you write about at least one thing you're thankful for that day.

9. The "More" section gives you additional room to write freestyle—expressing additional thoughts, expanding on details from previous sections, capturing the aha moments of the day, or simply reflecting on, or venting about, whatever you want or need to say.

10. For quick reference to your *Lupus Diary* entry pages by date, use the Table of Dates, found on page 13. After completing your diary entry, simply enter the date in the space provided next to its page number.

If you have questions, please feel free to contact me by e-mail at *olivia@lupusdiary.com* or by using the Contact form at *http://www.lupusdiary.com/contact/*.

The Live a Beautiful Life with Lupus Framework

The *Live a Beautiful Life with Lupus* framework is based on a list of habits and rituals that I believe help us thrive while living with this autoimmune disease. Below is a brief synopsis of the benefits of these habits and rituals, the goals of which are: 1) to soothe the Lupus body; 2) to strengthen the Lupus mind; and 3) to nurture the Lupus spirit. Each dimension of one's being—the body, mind, and spirit—integrally contribute and elevate the other, as shown in the framework diagram on page 12. To learn even more about how and why these habits and rituals support living well with Lupus, please refer to the book, *Live a Beautiful Life with Lupus*, shown on page 175.

Habits and rituals to soothe the Lupus body help to increase your body's ability to operate more efficiently by what you subject it to internally and externally.

- *Sleep Well* to get consistent, restful, restorative sleep to combat Lupus fatigue and help with overall healing.
- *Take a Warm Bath* to soothe painful muscles and joints.
- *Eat a Clean Diet* to maximize nutrition and minimize undesirable effects of a poor diet.
- *Move & Stretch* for gentle exercise that keeps mucles active and joints lubricated.
- *Breathe Fresh Air* to improve the cleansing action of the lungs and provide other oxygenating benefits.
- *Get a Gentle Massage* to help reduce inflammation and release pain-relieving endorphins.
- *Stay Hydrated* to avoid dehydration, which worsens inflammation and creates a burden on our organs.
- *Protect Delicate Skin* from the sun's harmful UV rays, which can cause Lupus flares and rashes.
- *Smile & Laugh* to gain benefits of humor therapy, including heart and lung oxygenation and pain-relieving endorphins.
- *Be Intimate* in personal relationships to reap the benefits of open communication and physical closeness—from hugs to sex.

Habits and rituals to strengthen the Lupus mind help you manage your emotions and behaviors so that you minimize Lupus flares, brain fog, and other mental manifestations of the disease.

- *Manage Expectations* of yourself and others, realizing that we all have limitations.
- *Manage Time & Energy* to minimize stress and help deal with brain fog and other cognitive issues caused by Lupus.
- *Ask For & Accept Help* to help meet responsibilities and demands, which are often adversely affected by Lupus.
- *Protect Alone Time* to help us become more in-tune with ourselves and replenish our over-worked minds.
- *Focus on the Positive* to see the proverbial glass as half-full, despite all that Lupus does to us.
- *Manage Stress Response* to prevent the negative effects of stress hormones released during a fight-or-flight reaction.

- *Forgive & Release* to let go of the emotional pain caused by our friends' and family's lack of understanding and poor response to our illness.
- *Learn About Lupus* to remain educated about what's happening with the disease in terms of research and treatment.
- *Connect with Your Doctor* to give him/her a true and honest account of how Lupus affects you; they need to know.

Habits and rituals to nurture the Lupus spirit help to develop a spiritual connection to maintain a positive effect on our health.

- *Enjoy Sacred Space*, a place where you are able to find peace and calm, indoors or outdoors, in a corner or an entire room.
- *Meditate, Pray, Visualize* to connect with your spiritual self, becoming centered and relaxed.
- *Cultivate Your Creativity* to express yourself through art, music, writing, or any other pursuit of beauty.
- *Make Someone Happy* with small gestures that reap the health benefits of giving and thinking of others.
- *Embrace Uncertainty* to transcend the fear of the unknown by accepting that nothing is certain in life.
- *Find and Live Your Purpose* to find happiness and inspiration in learning what you are meant to do and be in this life.
- *Love Yourself* to unconditionally accept yourself—someone living with Lupus—as lovable and worthy of self-compassion and self-respect.

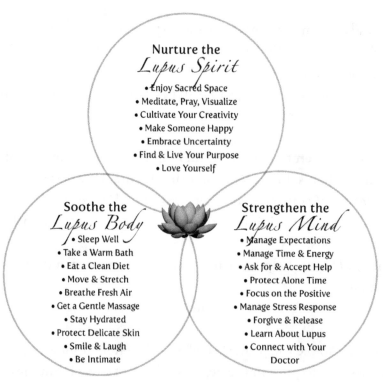

Nurture the
Lupus Spirit
• Enjoy Sacred Space
• Meditate, Pray, Visualize
• Cultivate Your Creativity
• Make Someone Happy
• Embrace Uncertainty
• Find & Live Your Purpose
• Love Yourself

Soothe the
Lupus Body
• Sleep Well
• Take a Warm Bath
• Eat a Clean Diet
• Move & Stretch
• Breathe Fresh Air
• Get a Gentle Massage
• Stay Hydrated
• Protect Delicate Skin
• Smile & Laugh
• Be Intimate

Strengthen the
Lupus Mind
• Manage Expectations
• Manage Time & Energy
• Ask for & Accept Help
• Protect Alone Time
• Focus on the Positive
• Manage Stress Response
• Forgive & Release
• Learn About Lupus
• Connect with Your Doctor

Diagram of the *Live a Beautiful Life with Lupus* Framework

Table of Lupus Diary Entry Dates

(For Quick Reference)

Today's Date: _____

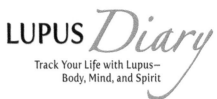

LUPUS *Diary*
Track Your Life with Lupus—
Body, Mind, and Spirit

Body

Today's Habits/Rituals to Soothe My Lupus Body:

○ *Slept Well*   ○ *Ate a Clean Diet*   ○ *Got a Gentle Massage*   ○ *Stayed Hydrated*   ○ *Smiled & Laughed*

○ *Took a Warm Bath*   ○ *Moved & Stretched*   ○ *Breathed Fresh Air*   ○ *Protected Skin*   ○ *Was Intimate*

Details and Thoughts About My Physical Symptoms Today:

_____

_____

_____

_____

Mind

Today's Habits/Rituals to Strengthen My Lupus Mind:

○ *Managed Expectations*   ○ *Asked for & Accepted Help*   ○ *Focused on the Positive*   ○ *Forgave & Released*   ○ *Connected with My Doctor*

○ *Managed Time & Energy*   ○ *Protected Alone Time*   ○ *Managed Stress Response*   ○ *Learned About Lupus*

Details and Thoughts About My Emotions Today:

_____

_____

_____

_____

Spirit

Today's Habits/Rituals to Nurture My Lupus Spirit:

○ *Enjoyed Sacred Space*   ○ *Cultivated Creativity*   ○ *Embraced Uncertainty*   ○ *Loved Myself*

○ *Meditated, Prayed, Visualized*   ○ *Made Someone Happy*   ○ *Worked on Finding and Living My Purpose*

Details and Thoughts About My Spiritual Connection Today:

_____

_____

_____

_____

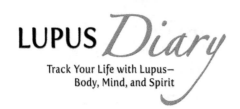

Meals

Breakfast	Lunch	Dinner
_____	_____	_____
_____	_____	_____
_____	_____	_____
_____	_____	_____

Snacks	Water	Reactions to Foods
_____	_____	_____
_____	_____	_____
_____	_____	_____
_____	_____	_____

Notes and Reminders

Items to remember to share with my doctor or other practitioner

_____

_____

_____

_____

_____

_____

_____

_____

_____

_____

_____

Today's Date:_____

LUPUS *Diary*

Track Your Life with Lupus—
Body, Mind, and Spirit

Gratitude

What am I thankful for today?

_____
_____
_____
_____
_____
_____
_____

More

More thoughts, details, feelings, aha moments about living with Lupus....

_____
_____
_____
_____
_____
_____
_____
_____
_____
_____
_____
_____
_____
_____
_____
_____
_____

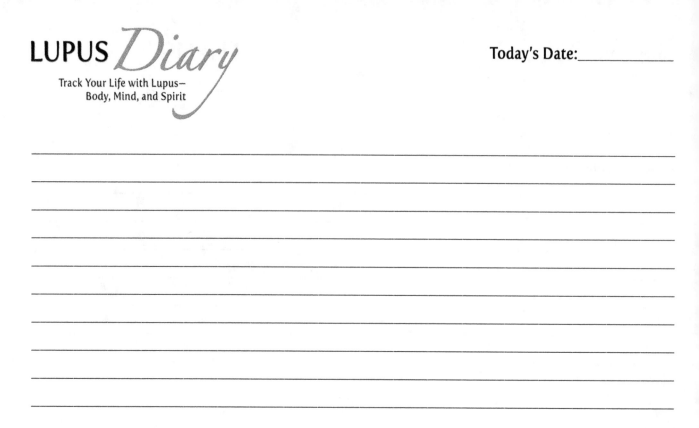

LUPUS *Diary*

Track Your Life with Lupus—
Body, Mind, and Spirit

Today's Date:_____

_____
_____
_____
_____
_____
_____
_____
_____
_____
_____
_____
_____
_____
_____
_____
_____

The lotus comes from the murkiest water, but grows into the purest thing.

Nita Ambani

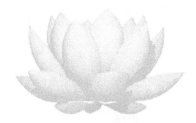

Today's Date:_____

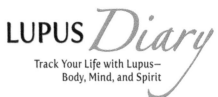

LUPUS Diary
Track Your Life with Lupus—
Body, Mind, and Spirit

Body

Today's Habits/Rituals to Soothe My Lupus Body:

○ *Slept Well*   ○ *Ate a Clean Diet*   ○ *Got a Gentle Massage*   ○ *Stayed Hydrated*   ○ *Smiled & Laughed*
○ *Took a Warm Bath*   ○ *Moved & Stretched*   ○ *Breathed Fresh Air*   ○ *Protected Skin*   ○ *Was Intimate*

Details and Thoughts About My Physical Symptoms Today:

_____

_____

_____

_____

Mind

Today's Habits/Rituals to Strengthen My Lupus Mind:

○ *Managed Expectations*   ○ *Asked for & Accepted Help*   ○ *Focused on the Positive*   ○ *Forgave & Released*   ○ *Connected with My Doctor*
○ *Managed Time & Energy*   ○ *Protected Alone Time*   ○ *Managed Stress Response*   ○ *Learned About Lupus*

Details and Thoughts About My Emotions Today:

_____

_____

_____

_____

Spirit

Today's Habits/Rituals to Nurture My Lupus Spirit:

○ *Enjoyed Sacred Space*   ○ *Cultivated Creativity*   ○ *Embraced Uncertainty*   ○ *Loved Myself*
○ *Meditated, Prayed, Visualized*   ○ *Made Someone Happy*   ○ *Worked on Finding and Living My Purpose*

Details and Thoughts About My Spiritual Connection Today:

_____

_____

_____

_____

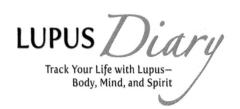 **LUPUS** *Diary*

Track Your Life with Lupus—
Body, Mind, and Spirit

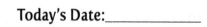

Meals

Breakfast	Lunch	Dinner
_____	_____	_____
_____	_____	_____
_____	_____	_____
_____	_____	_____

Snacks	Water	Reactions to Foods
_____	_____	_____
_____	_____	_____
_____	_____	_____
_____	_____	_____

Notes and Reminders

Items to remember to share with my doctor or other practitioner

Today's Date:_____

LUPUS *Diary*

Track Your Life with Lupus—
Body, Mind, and Spirit

Gratitude

What am I thankful for today?

_____

_____

_____

_____

_____

_____

_____

More

More thoughts, details, feelings, aha moments about living with Lupus....

_____

_____

_____

_____

_____

_____

_____

_____

_____

_____

_____

_____

_____

_____

_____

_____

_____

LUPUS *Diary*

Track Your Life with Lupus—
Body, Mind, and Spirit

_____

_____

_____

_____

_____

_____

_____

_____

_____

_____

_____

_____

_____

_____

_____

_____

*Guard your mental house so
that no negative thoughts
find entrance.*

Unknown

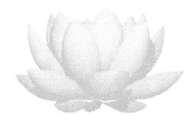

Today's Date:_____

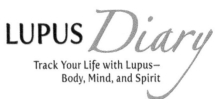

LUPUS *Diary*

Track Your Life with Lupus—
Body, Mind, and Spirit

Body

Today's Habits/Rituals to Soothe My Lupus Body:

○ *Slept Well*   ○ *Ate a Clean Diet*   ○ *Got a Gentle Massage*   ○ *Stayed Hydrated*   ○ *Smiled & Laughed*

○ *Took a Warm Bath*   ○ *Moved & Stretched*   ○ *Breathed Fresh Air*   ○ *Protected Skin*   ○ *Was Intimate*

Details and Thoughts About My Physical Symptoms Today:

_____

_____

_____

_____

Mind

Today's Habits/Rituals to Strengthen My Lupus Mind:

○ *Managed Expectations*   ○ *Asked for & Accepted Help*   ○ *Focused on the Positive*   ○ *Forgave & Released*   ○ *Connected with My Doctor*

○ *Managed Time & Energy*   ○ *Protected Alone Time*   ○ *Managed Stress Response*   ○ *Learned About Lupus*

Details and Thoughts About My Emotions Today:

_____

_____

_____

_____

Spirit

Today's Habits/Rituals to Nurture My Lupus Spirit:

○ *Enjoyed Sacred Space*   ○ *Cultivated Creativity*   ○ *Embraced Uncertainty*   ○ *Loved Myself*

○ *Meditated, Prayed, Visualized*   ○ *Made Someone Happy*   ○ *Worked on Finding and Living My Purpose*

Details and Thoughts About My Spiritual Connection Today:

_____

_____

_____

_____

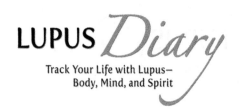 # LUPUS *Diary*

Track Your Life with Lupus—
Body, Mind, and Spirit

Meals

Breakfast

_____
_____
_____
_____

Lunch

_____
_____
_____
_____

Dinner

_____
_____
_____
_____

Snacks

_____
_____
_____
_____

Water

_____
_____
_____
_____

Reactions to Foods

_____
_____
_____
_____

Notes and Reminders

Items to remember to share with my doctor or other practitioner

_____
_____
_____
_____
_____
_____
_____
_____
_____
_____
_____
_____

Today's Date:_____

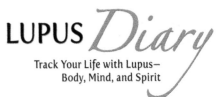

Gratitude

What am I thankful for today?

_____

_____

_____

_____

_____

_____

_____

More

More thoughts, details, feelings, aha moments about living with Lupus....

_____

_____

_____

_____

_____

_____

_____

_____

_____

_____

_____

_____

_____

_____

_____

_____

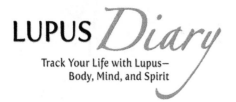

LUPUS *Diary*

Track Your Life with Lupus—
Body, Mind, and Spirit

_____

_____

_____

_____

_____

_____

_____

_____

_____

_____

_____

_____

_____

_____

_____

_____

Life shrinks or expands in proportion to one's courage.

Anais Nin

Today's Date:_____

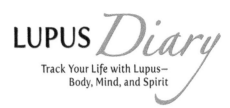

Body

Today's Habits/Rituals to Soothe My Lupus Body:

○ Slept Well   ○ Ate a Clean Diet   ○ Got a Gentle Massage   ○ Stayed Hydrated   ○ Smiled & Laughed

○ Took a Warm Bath   ○ Moved & Stretched   ○ Breathed Fresh Air   ○ Protected Skin   ○ Was Intimate

Details and Thoughts About My Physical Symptoms Today:

_____

_____

_____

_____

Mind

Today's Habits/Rituals to Strengthen My Lupus Mind:

○ Managed Expectations   ○ Asked for & Accepted Help   ○ Focused on the Positive   ○ Forgave & Released   ○ Connected with My Doctor

○ Managed Time & Energy   ○ Protected Alone Time   ○ Managed Stress Response   ○ Learned About Lupus

Details and Thoughts About My Emotions Today:

_____

_____

_____

_____

Spirit

Today's Habits/Rituals to Nurture My Lupus Spirit:

○ Enjoyed Sacred Space   ○ Cultivated Creativity   ○ Embraced Uncertainty   ○ Loved Myself

○ Meditated, Prayed, Visualized   ○ Made Someone Happy   ○ Worked on Finding and Living My Purpose

Details and Thoughts About My Spiritual Connection Today:

_____

_____

_____

_____

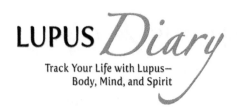 LUPUS *Diary*

Track Your Life with Lupus—
Body, Mind, and Spirit

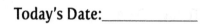

Meals

Breakfast

_____
_____
_____
_____

Lunch

_____
_____
_____
_____

Dinner

_____
_____
_____
_____

Snacks

_____
_____
_____
_____

Water

_____
_____
_____
_____

Reactions to Foods

_____
_____
_____
_____

Notes and Reminders

Items to remember to share with my doctor or other practitioner

_____
_____
_____
_____
_____
_____
_____
_____
_____
_____
_____
_____

Today's Date:_____

Gratitude

What am I thankful for today?

_____

_____

_____

_____

_____

_____

More

More thoughts, details, feelings, aha moments about living with Lupus....

_____

_____

_____

_____

_____

_____

_____

_____

_____

_____

_____

_____

_____

_____

LUPUS *Diary*

Track Your Life with Lupus—
Body, Mind, and Spirit

_____

_____

_____

_____

_____

_____

_____

_____

_____

_____

_____

_____

_____

_____

_____

*Medicine is a science of
uncertainty and
an art of probability.*

William Osler

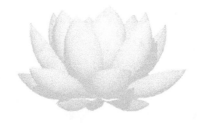

Today's Date:_____

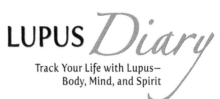

LUPUS *Diary*

Track Your Life with Lupus—
Body, Mind, and Spirit

Body

Today's Habits/Rituals to Soothe My Lupus Body:

○ *Slept Well*   ○ *Ate a Clean Diet*   ○ *Got a Gentle Massage*   ○ *Stayed Hydrated*   ○ *Smiled & Laughed*

○ *Took a Warm Bath*   ○ *Moved & Stretched*   ○ *Breathed Fresh Air*   ○ *Protected Skin*   ○ *Was Intimate*

Details and Thoughts About My Physical Symptoms Today:

_____

_____

_____

_____

Mind

Today's Habits/Rituals to Strengthen My Lupus Mind:

○ *Managed Expectations*   ○ *Asked for & Accepted Help*   ○ *Focused on the Positive*   ○ *Forgave & Released*   ○ *Connected*

○ *Managed Time & Energy*   ○ *Protected Alone Time*   ○ *Managed Stress Response*   ○ *Learned About Lupus*   *with My Doctor*

Details and Thoughts About My Emotions Today:

_____

_____

_____

_____

Spirit

Today's Habits/Rituals to Nurture My Lupus Spirit:

○ *Enjoyed Sacred Space*   ○ *Cultivated Creativity*   ○ *Embraced Uncertainty*   ○ *Loved Myself*

○ *Meditated, Prayed, Visualized* ○ *Made Someone Happy*   ○ *Worked on Finding and Living My Purpose*

Details and Thoughts About My Spiritual Connection Today:

_____

_____

_____

_____

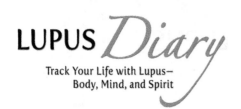
LUPUS *Diary*
Track Your Life with Lupus—
Body, Mind, and Spirit

Meals

Breakfast

_____

_____

_____

_____

Lunch

_____

_____

_____

_____

Dinner

_____

_____

_____

_____

Snacks

_____

_____

_____

_____

Water

_____

_____

_____

_____

Reactions to Foods

_____

_____

_____

_____

Notes and Reminders

Items to remember to share with my doctor or other practitioner

_____

_____

_____

_____

_____

_____

_____

_____

_____

_____

_____

Today's Date:_____

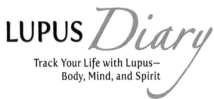

Gratitude

What am I thankful for today?

_____

_____

_____

_____

_____

_____

_____

More

More thoughts, details, feelings, aha moments about living with Lupus....

_____

_____

_____

_____

_____

_____

_____

_____

_____

_____

_____

_____

_____

_____

_____

_____

_____

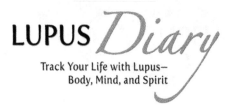

LUPUS *Diary*

Track Your Life with Lupus—
Body, Mind, and Spirit

Today's Date:_____

_____
_____
_____
_____
_____
_____
_____
_____
_____
_____
_____
_____
_____
_____
_____
_____
_____

Perseverance,
secret of all triumphs.

Victor Hugo

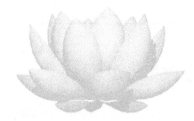

Today's Date:_____

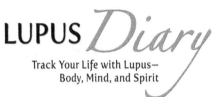

Body

Today's Habits/Rituals to Soothe My Lupus Body:

○ *Slept Well*　　　○ *Ate a Clean Diet*　　　○ *Got a Gentle Massage*　　　○ *Stayed Hydrated*　　　○ *Smiled & Laughed*

○ *Took a Warm Bath*　　○ *Moved & Stretched*　　○ *Breathed Fresh Air*　　○ *Protected Skin*　　○ *Was Intimate*

Details and Thoughts About My Physical Symptoms Today:

_____

_____

_____

_____

Mind

Today's Habits/Rituals to Strengthen My Lupus Mind:

○ *Managed Expectations*　○ *Asked for & Accepted Help*　○ *Focused on the Positive*　○ *Forgave & Released*　○ *Connected with My Doctor*

○ *Managed Time & Energy*　○ *Protected Alone Time*　　○ *Managed Stress Response*　○ *Learned About Lupus*

Details and Thoughts About My Emotions Today:

_____

_____

_____

_____

Spirit

Today's Habits/Rituals to Nurture My Lupus Spirit:

○ *Enjoyed Sacred Space*　　　○ *Cultivated Creativity*　　　○ *Embraced Uncertainty*　　　○ *Loved Myself*

○ *Meditated, Prayed, Visualized*　　○ *Made Someone Happy*　　○ *Worked on Finding and Living My Purpose*

Details and Thoughts About My Spiritual Connection Today:

_____

_____

_____

_____

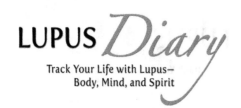

Meals

Breakfast	Lunch	Dinner
_____	_____	_____
_____	_____	_____
_____	_____	_____
_____	_____	_____

Snacks	Water	Reactions to Foods
_____	_____	_____
_____	_____	_____
_____	_____	_____
_____	_____	_____

Notes and Reminders

Items to remember to share with my doctor or other practitioner

_____

_____

_____

_____

_____

_____

_____

_____

_____

_____

_____

Today's Date:_____

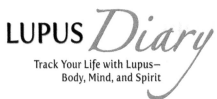

LUPUS *Diary*
Track Your Life with Lupus—
Body, Mind, and Spirit

Gratitude

What am I thankful for today?

_____

_____

_____

_____

_____

_____

_____

More

More thoughts, details, feelings, aha moments about living with Lupus....

_____

_____

_____

_____

_____

_____

_____

_____

_____

_____

_____

_____

_____

_____

_____

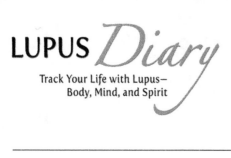

LUPUS *Diary*

Track Your Life with Lupus—
Body, Mind, and Spirit

Today's Date:_____

_____

_____

_____

_____

_____

_____

_____

_____

_____

_____

_____

_____

_____

_____

_____

_____

_____

*Your sacred space is where
you can find yourself
again and again.*

Joseph Campbell

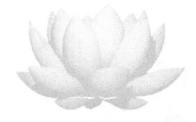

Today's Date:_____

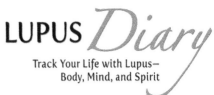

Body

Today's Habits/Rituals to Soothe My Lupus Body:

○ *Slept Well*   ○ *Ate a Clean Diet*   ○ *Got a Gentle Massage*   ○ *Stayed Hydrated*   ○ *Smiled & Laughed*

○ *Took a Warm Bath*   ○ *Moved & Stretched*   ○ *Breathed Fresh Air*   ○ *Protected Skin*   ○ *Was Intimate*

Details and Thoughts About My Physical Symptoms Today:

_____

_____

_____

_____

Mind

Today's Habits/Rituals to Strengthen My Lupus Mind:

○ *Managed Expectations*   ○ *Asked for & Accepted Help*   ○ *Focused on the Positive*   ○ *Forgave & Released*   ○ *Connected*

○ *Managed Time & Energy*   ○ *Protected Alone Time*   ○ *Managed Stress Response*   ○ *Learned About Lupus*   *with My Doctor*

Details and Thoughts About My Emotions Today:

_____

_____

_____

_____

Spirit

Today's Habits/Rituals to Nurture My Lupus Spirit:

○ *Enjoyed Sacred Space*   ○ *Cultivated Creativity*   ○ *Embraced Uncertainty*   ○ *Loved Myself*

○ *Meditated, Prayed, Visualized*   ○ *Made Someone Happy*   ○ *Worked on Finding and Living My Purpose*

Details and Thoughts About My Spiritual Connection Today:

_____

_____

_____

_____

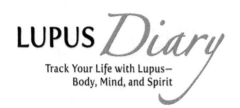

LUPUS *Diary*

Track Your Life with Lupus—
Body, Mind, and Spirit

Meals

Breakfast

_____
_____
_____
_____

Lunch

_____
_____
_____
_____

Dinner

_____
_____
_____
_____

Snacks

_____
_____
_____
_____

Water

_____
_____
_____
_____

Reactions to Foods

_____
_____
_____
_____

Notes and Reminders

Items to remember to share with my doctor or other practitioner

_____
_____
_____
_____
_____
_____
_____
_____
_____
_____
_____

Today's Date:_____

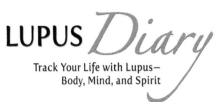

LUPUS *Diary*
Track Your Life with Lupus—
Body, Mind, and Spirit

Gratitude

What am I thankful for today?

_____

_____

_____

_____

_____

_____

_____

More

More thoughts, details, feelings, aha moments about living with Lupus....

_____

_____

_____

_____

_____

_____

_____

_____

_____

_____

_____

_____

_____

_____

_____

_____

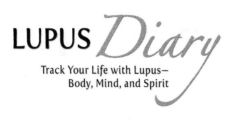

LUPUS *Diary*

Track Your Life with Lupus—
Body, Mind, and Spirit

Today's Date:_____

_____

_____

_____

_____

_____

_____

_____

_____

_____

_____

_____

_____

_____

_____

_____

I am grateful for what I am and have.
My thanksgiving is perpetual.

Henry David Thoreau

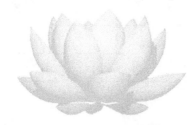

Today's Date:_____

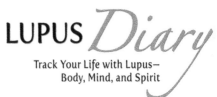

LUPUS *Diary*

Track Your Life with Lupus—
Body, Mind, and Spirit

Body

Today's Habits/Rituals to Soothe My Lupus Body:

○ *Slept Well*   ○ *Ate a Clean Diet*   ○ *Got a Gentle Massage*   ○ *Stayed Hydrated*   ○ *Smiled & Laughed*

○ *Took a Warm Bath*   ○ *Moved & Stretched*   ○ *Breathed Fresh Air*   ○ *Protected Skin*   ○ *Was Intimate*

Details and Thoughts About My Physical Symptoms Today:

_____

_____

_____

_____

Mind

Today's Habits/Rituals to Strengthen My Lupus Mind:

○ *Managed Expectations*   ○ *Asked for & Accepted Help* ○ *Focused on the Positive*   ○ *Forgave & Released*   ○ *Connected*

○ *Managed Time & Energy* ○ *Protected Alone Time*   ○ *Managed Stress Response* ○ *Learned About Lupus*   *with My Doctor*

Details and Thoughts About My Emotions Today:

_____

_____

_____

_____

Spirit

Today's Habits/Rituals to Nurture My Lupus Spirit:

○ *Enjoyed Sacred Space*   ○ *Cultivated Creativity*   ○ *Embraced Uncertainty*   ○ *Loved Myself*

○ *Meditated, Prayed, Visualized*   ○ *Made Someone Happy*   ○ *Worked on Finding and Living My Purpose*

Details and Thoughts About My Spiritual Connection Today:

_____

_____

_____

_____

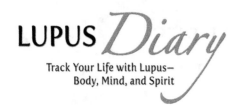

LUPUS *Diary*

Track Your Life with Lupus—
Body, Mind, and Spirit

Meals

Breakfast

_____
_____
_____
_____

Lunch

_____
_____
_____
_____

Dinner

_____
_____
_____
_____

Snacks

_____
_____
_____

Water

_____
_____
_____

Reactions to Foods

_____
_____
_____

Notes and Reminders

Items to remember to share with my doctor or other practitioner

_____
_____
_____
_____
_____
_____
_____
_____
_____
_____

Today's Date:_____

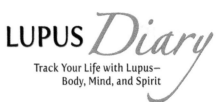

Gratitude

What am I thankful for today?

_____
_____
_____
_____
_____
_____

More

More thoughts, details, feelings, aha moments about living with Lupus....

_____
_____
_____
_____
_____
_____
_____
_____
_____
_____
_____
_____
_____
_____
_____

LUPUS *Diary*

Track Your Life with Lupus—
Body, Mind, and Spirit

_____

_____

_____

_____

_____

_____

_____

_____

_____

_____

_____

_____

_____

_____

_____

_____

_____

*When you reach the end of
your rope, tie a knot in it
and hang on.*

Franklin D. Roosevelt

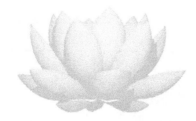

Today's Date:_____

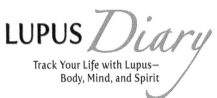

Body

Today's Habits/Rituals to Soothe My Lupus Body:

○ *Slept Well*　　　○ *Ate a Clean Diet*　　　○ *Got a Gentle Massage*　　　○ *Stayed Hydrated*　　　○ *Smiled & Laughed*

○ *Took a Warm Bath*　　○ *Moved & Stretched*　　○ *Breathed Fresh Air*　　○ *Protected Skin*　　○ *Was Intimate*

Details and Thoughts About My Physical Symptoms Today:

_____

_____

_____

_____

Mind

Today's Habits/Rituals to Strengthen My Lupus Mind:

○ *Managed Expectations*　　○ *Asked for & Accepted Help*　　○ *Focused on the Positive*　　○ *Forgave & Released*　　○ *Connected with My Doctor*

○ *Managed Time & Energy*　　○ *Protected Alone Time*　　○ *Managed Stress Response*　　○ *Learned About Lupus*

Details and Thoughts About My Emotions Today:

_____

_____

_____

_____

Spirit

Today's Habits/Rituals to Nurture My Lupus Spirit:

○ *Enjoyed Sacred Space*　　○ *Cultivated Creativity*　　○ *Embraced Uncertainty*　　○ *Loved Myself*

○ *Meditated, Prayed, Visualized*　　○ *Made Someone Happy*　　○ *Worked on Finding and Living My Purpose*

Details and Thoughts About My Spiritual Connection Today:

_____

_____

_____

_____

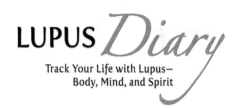 **LUPUS** *Diary*

Track Your Life with Lupus—
Body, Mind, and Spirit

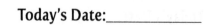 **Today's Date:**_____

Meals

Breakfast	Lunch	Dinner
_____	_____	_____
_____	_____	_____
_____	_____	_____
_____	_____	_____

Snacks	Water	Reactions to Foods
_____	_____	_____
_____	_____	_____
_____	_____	_____

Notes and Reminders

Items to remember to share with my doctor or other practitioner

_____

_____

_____

_____

_____

_____

_____

_____

_____

_____

Today's Date:_____

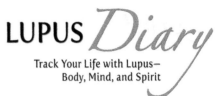

Gratitude

What am I thankful for today?

_____

_____

_____

_____

_____

_____

_____

More

More thoughts, details, feelings, aha moments about living with Lupus....

_____

_____

_____

_____

_____

_____

_____

_____

_____

_____

_____

_____

_____

_____

LUPUS *Diary*
Track Your Life with Lupus—
Body, Mind, and Spirit

_____

_____

_____

_____

_____

_____

_____

_____

_____

_____

_____

_____

_____

_____

_____

_____

*What lies behind you and what lies in front
of you, pales in comparison to
what lies inside of you.*

Ralph Waldo Emerson

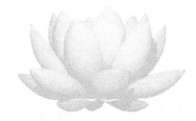

Today's Date:_____

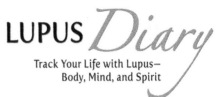

Body

Today's Habits/Rituals to Soothe My Lupus Body:

○ Slept Well   ○ Ate a Clean Diet   ○ Got a Gentle Massage   ○ Stayed Hydrated   ○ Smiled & Laughed

○ Took a Warm Bath   ○ Moved & Stretched   ○ Breathed Fresh Air   ○ Protected Skin   ○ Was Intimate

Details and Thoughts About My Physical Symptoms Today:

_____

_____

_____

_____

Mind

Today's Habits/Rituals to Strengthen My Lupus Mind:

○ Managed Expectations   ○ Asked for & Accepted Help   ○ Focused on the Positive   ○ Forgave & Released   ○ Connected with My Doctor

○ Managed Time & Energy   ○ Protected Alone Time   ○ Managed Stress Response   ○ Learned About Lupus

Details and Thoughts About My Emotions Today:

_____

_____

_____

_____

Spirit

Today's Habits/Rituals to Nurture My Lupus Spirit:

○ Enjoyed Sacred Space   ○ Cultivated Creativity   ○ Embraced Uncertainty   ○ Loved Myself

○ Meditated, Prayed, Visualized   ○ Made Someone Happy   ○ Worked on Finding and Living My Purpose

Details and Thoughts About My Spiritual Connection Today:

_____

_____

_____

_____

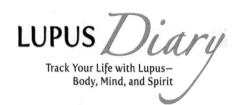LUPUS *Diary*

Track Your Life with Lupus—
Body, Mind, and Spirit

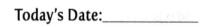**Today's Date:**_____

Meals

Breakfast

_____

_____

_____

_____

Lunch

_____

_____

_____

_____

Dinner

_____

_____

_____

_____

Snacks

_____

_____

_____

_____

Water

_____

_____

_____

_____

Reactions to Foods

_____

_____

_____

_____

Notes and Reminders

Items to remember to share with my doctor or other practitioner

_____

_____

_____

_____

_____

_____

_____

_____

_____

_____

_____

Today's Date:_____

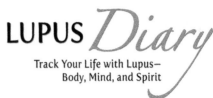

Gratitude

What am I thankful for today?

_____

_____

_____

_____

_____

_____

_____

More

More thoughts, details, feelings, aha moments about living with Lupus....

_____

_____

_____

_____

_____

_____

_____

_____

_____

_____

_____

_____

_____

_____

_____

_____

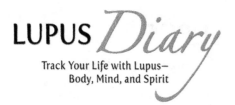
LUPUS *Diary*
Track Your Life with Lupus—
Body, Mind, and Spirit

_____
_____
_____
_____
_____
_____
_____
_____
_____
_____
_____
_____
_____
_____
_____
_____

Perhaps I am stronger than I think.

Thomas Merton

Today's Date:_____

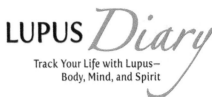

LUPUS *Diary*

Track Your Life with Lupus—
Body, Mind, and Spirit

Body

Today's Habits/Rituals to Soothe My Lupus Body:

○ *Slept Well*　　　○ *Ate a Clean Diet*　　　○ *Got a Gentle Massage*　　　○ *Stayed Hydrated*　　　○ *Smiled & Laughed*

○ *Took a Warm Bath*　　○ *Moved & Stretched*　　○ *Breathed Fresh Air*　　○ *Protected Skin*　　○ *Was Intimate*

Details and Thoughts About My Physical Symptoms Today:

_____

_____

_____

_____

Mind

Today's Habits/Rituals to Strengthen My Lupus Mind:

○ *Managed Expectations*　○ *Asked for & Accepted Help*　○ *Focused on the Positive*　○ *Forgave & Released*　○ *Connected with My Doctor*

○ *Managed Time & Energy*　○ *Protected Alone Time*　　○ *Managed Stress Response*　○ *Learned About Lupus*

Details and Thoughts About My Emotions Today:

_____

_____

_____

_____

Spirit

Today's Habits/Rituals to Nurture My Lupus Spirit:

○ *Enjoyed Sacred Space*　　　○ *Cultivated Creativity*　　　○ *Embraced Uncertainty*　　　○ *Loved Myself*

○ *Meditated, Prayed, Visualized*　　○ *Made Someone Happy*　　○ *Worked on Finding and Living My Purpose*

Details and Thoughts About My Spiritual Connection Today:

_____

_____

_____

_____

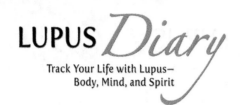 **LUPUS** *Diary*

Track Your Life with Lupus—
Body, Mind, and Spirit

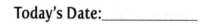 **Today's Date:**_____

Meals

Breakfast

_____

_____

_____

_____

Lunch

_____

_____

_____

_____

Dinner

_____

_____

_____

_____

Snacks

_____

_____

_____

_____

Water

_____

_____

_____

_____

Reactions to Foods

_____

_____

_____

_____

Notes and Reminders

Items to remember to share with my doctor or other practitioner

_____

_____

_____

_____

_____

_____

_____

_____

_____

_____

_____

Today's Date:_____

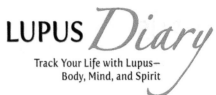

LUPUS *Diary*

Track Your Life with Lupus—
Body, Mind, and Spirit

Gratitude

What am I thankful for today?

_____

_____

_____

_____

_____

_____

_____

More

More thoughts, details, feelings, aha moments about living with Lupus....

_____

_____

_____

_____

_____

_____

_____

_____

_____

_____

_____

_____

_____

_____

_____

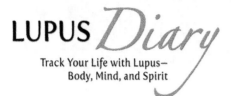
_____

_____

_____

_____

_____

_____

_____

_____

_____

_____

_____

_____

_____

_____

_____

_____

*I'm not afraid of storms, for I'm
learning how to sail my ship.*

Louisa May Alcott

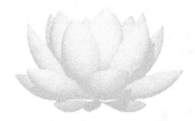

Today's Date:_____

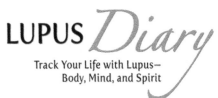

LUPUS *Diary*

Track Your Life with Lupus—
Body, Mind, and Spirit

Body

Today's Habits/Rituals to Soothe My Lupus Body:

○ Slept Well   ○ Ate a Clean Diet   ○ Got a Gentle Massage   ○ Stayed Hydrated   ○ Smiled & Laughed

○ Took a Warm Bath   ○ Moved & Stretched   ○ Breathed Fresh Air   ○ Protected Skin   ○ Was Intimate

Details and Thoughts About My Physical Symptoms Today:

_____

_____

_____

_____

Mind

Today's Habits/Rituals to Strengthen My Lupus Mind:

○ Managed Expectations   ○ Asked for & Accepted Help   ○ Focused on the Positive   ○ Forgave & Released   ○ Connected with My Doctor

○ Managed Time & Energy   ○ Protected Alone Time   ○ Managed Stress Response   ○ Learned About Lupus

Details and Thoughts About My Emotions Today:

_____

_____

_____

_____

Spirit

Today's Habits/Rituals to Nurture My Lupus Spirit:

○ Enjoyed Sacred Space   ○ Cultivated Creativity   ○ Embraced Uncertainty   ○ Loved Myself

○ Meditated, Prayed, Visualized   ○ Made Someone Happy   ○ Worked on Finding and Living My Purpose

Details and Thoughts About My Spiritual Connection Today:

_____

_____

_____

_____

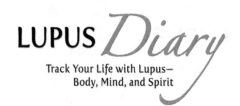
LUPUS *Diary*

Track Your Life with Lupus—
Body, Mind, and Spirit

Meals

Breakfast	Lunch	Dinner
_____	_____	_____
_____	_____	_____
_____	_____	_____
_____	_____	_____

Snacks	Water	Reactions to Foods
_____	_____	_____
_____	_____	_____
_____	_____	_____
_____	_____	_____

Notes and Reminders

Items to remember to share with my doctor or other practitioner

_____
_____
_____
_____
_____
_____
_____
_____
_____
_____
_____

Today's Date:_____

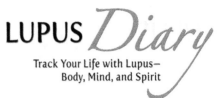

Gratitude

What am I thankful for today?

_____

_____

_____

_____

_____

_____

_____

More

More thoughts, details, feelings, aha moments about living with Lupus....

_____

_____

_____

_____

_____

_____

_____

_____

_____

_____

_____

_____

_____

_____

_____

_____

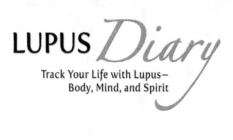

Today's Date:_____

_____
_____
_____
_____
_____
_____
_____
_____
_____
_____
_____
_____
_____
_____
_____
_____
_____

*When the mind, body, and spirit
work together, I believe
anything is possible.*

Criss Angel

Today's Date:_____

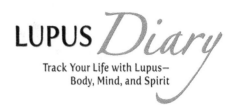

LUPUS *Diary*
Track Your Life with Lupus—
Body, Mind, and Spirit

Body

Today's Habits/Rituals to Soothe My Lupus Body:

○ *Slept Well*   ○ *Ate a Clean Diet*   ○ *Got a Gentle Massage*   ○ *Stayed Hydrated*   ○ *Smiled & Laughed*

○ *Took a Warm Bath*   ○ *Moved & Stretched*   ○ *Breathed Fresh Air*   ○ *Protected Skin*   ○ *Was Intimate*

Details and Thoughts About My Physical Symptoms Today:

_____

_____

_____

_____

Mind

Today's Habits/Rituals to Strengthen My Lupus Mind:

○ *Managed Expectations*   ○ *Asked for & Accepted Help*   ○ *Focused on the Positive*   ○ *Forgave & Released*   ○ *Connected with My Doctor*

○ *Managed Time & Energy*   ○ *Protected Alone Time*   ○ *Managed Stress Response*   ○ *Learned About Lupus*

Details and Thoughts About My Emotions Today:

_____

_____

_____

_____

Spirit

Today's Habits/Rituals to Nurture My Lupus Spirit:

○ *Enjoyed Sacred Space*   ○ *Cultivated Creativity*   ○ *Embraced Uncertainty*   ○ *Loved Myself*

○ *Meditated, Prayed, Visualized*   ○ *Made Someone Happy*   ○ *Worked on Finding and Living My Purpose*

Details and Thoughts About My Spiritual Connection Today:

_____

_____

_____

_____

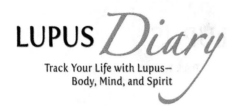

Meals

Breakfast	Lunch	Dinner
_____	_____	_____
_____	_____	_____
_____	_____	_____
_____	_____	_____

Snacks	Water	Reactions to Foods
_____	_____	_____
_____	_____	_____
_____	_____	_____

Notes and Reminders

Items to remember to share with my doctor or other practitioner

_____

_____

_____

_____

_____

_____

_____

_____

_____

_____

Today's Date:_____

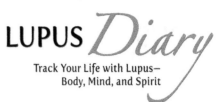

LUPUS *Diary*

Track Your Life with Lupus—
Body, Mind, and Spirit

Gratitude

What am I thankful for today?

_____

_____

_____

_____

_____

_____

_____

More

More thoughts, details, feelings, aha moments about living with Lupus....

_____

_____

_____

_____

_____

_____

_____

_____

_____

_____

_____

_____

_____

_____

_____

_____

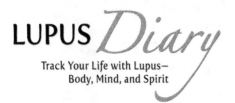
_____

_____

_____

_____

_____

_____

_____

_____

_____

_____

_____

_____

_____

_____

_____

_____

_____

*The part can never be well
unless the whole is well.*

Plato

Today's Date:_____

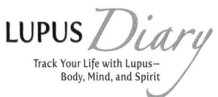

LUPUS *Diary*

Track Your Life with Lupus—
Body, Mind, and Spirit

Body

Today's Habits/Rituals to Soothe My Lupus Body:

○ Slept Well   ○ Ate a Clean Diet   ○ Got a Gentle Massage   ○ Stayed Hydrated   ○ Smiled & Laughed
○ Took a Warm Bath   ○ Moved & Stretched   ○ Breathed Fresh Air   ○ Protected Skin   ○ Was Intimate

Details and Thoughts About My Physical Symptoms Today:

_____

_____

_____

_____

Mind

Today's Habits/Rituals to Strengthen My Lupus Mind:

○ Managed Expectations   ○ Asked for & Accepted Help ○ Focused on the Positive   ○ Forgave & Released   ○ Connected
○ Managed Time & Energy   ○ Protected Alone Time   ○ Managed Stress Response   ○ Learned About Lupus   with My
                                                                                                              Doctor

Details and Thoughts About My Emotions Today:

_____

_____

_____

_____

Spirit

Today's Habits/Rituals to Nurture My Lupus Spirit:

○ Enjoyed Sacred Space   ○ Cultivated Creativity   ○ Embraced Uncertainty   ○ Loved Myself
○ Meditated, Prayed, Visualized ○ Made Someone Happy   ○ Worked on Finding and Living My Purpose

Details and Thoughts About My Spiritual Connection Today:

_____

_____

_____

_____

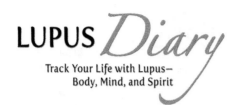

LUPUS *Diary*

Track Your Life with Lupus—
Body, Mind, and Spirit

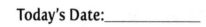

Today's Date:_____

Meals

Breakfast

_____

_____

_____

_____

Lunch

_____

_____

_____

_____

Dinner

_____

_____

_____

_____

Snacks

_____

_____

_____

_____

Water

_____

_____

_____

_____

Reactions to Foods

_____

_____

_____

_____

Notes and Reminders

Items to remember to share with my doctor or other practitioner

_____

_____

_____

_____

_____

_____

_____

_____

_____

_____

Today's Date:_____

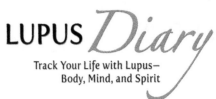

LUPUS *Diary*
Track Your Life with Lupus—
Body, Mind, and Spirit

Gratitude

What am I thankful for today?

_____

_____

_____

_____

_____

_____

_____

More

More thoughts, details, feelings, aha moments about living with Lupus....

_____

_____

_____

_____

_____

_____

_____

_____

_____

_____

_____

_____

_____

_____

_____

_____

_____

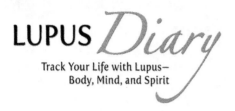

LUPUS *Diary*

Track Your Life with Lupus—
Body, Mind, and Spirit

_____
_____
_____
_____
_____
_____
_____
_____
_____
_____
_____
_____
_____
_____
_____
_____

*Let food be thy medicine and
medicine be thy food.*

Hippocrates

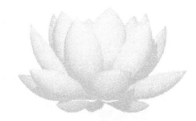

Today's Date:_____

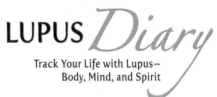

LUPUS *Diary*

Track Your Life with Lupus—
Body, Mind, and Spirit

Body

Today's Habits/Rituals to Soothe My Lupus Body:

○ Slept Well ○ Ate a Clean Diet ○ Got a Gentle Massage ○ Stayed Hydrated ○ Smiled & Laughed

○ Took a Warm Bath ○ Moved & Stretched ○ Breathed Fresh Air ○ Protected Skin ○ Was Intimate

Details and Thoughts About My Physical Symptoms Today:

_____

_____

_____

_____

Mind

Today's Habits/Rituals to Strengthen My Lupus Mind:

○ Managed Expectations ○ Asked for & Accepted Help ○ Focused on the Positive ○ Forgave & Released ○ Connected with My Doctor

○ Managed Time & Energy ○ Protected Alone Time ○ Managed Stress Response ○ Learned About Lupus

Details and Thoughts About My Emotions Today:

_____

_____

_____

_____

Spirit

Today's Habits/Rituals to Nurture My Lupus Spirit:

○ Enjoyed Sacred Space ○ Cultivated Creativity ○ Embraced Uncertainty ○ Loved Myself

○ Meditated, Prayed, Visualized ○ Made Someone Happy ○ Worked on Finding and Living My Purpose

Details and Thoughts About My Spiritual Connection Today:

_____

_____

_____

_____

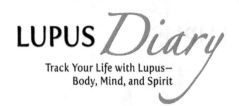 **LUPUS** *Diary*

Track Your Life with Lupus—
Body, Mind, and Spirit

 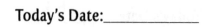

Meals

Breakfast

_____
_____
_____
_____

Lunch

_____
_____
_____
_____

Dinner

_____
_____
_____
_____

Snacks

_____
_____
_____
_____

Water

_____
_____
_____
_____

Reactions to Foods

_____
_____
_____
_____

Notes and Reminders

Items to remember to share with my doctor or other practitioner

_____
_____
_____
_____
_____
_____
_____
_____
_____
_____
_____
_____

Today's Date:_____

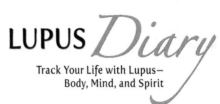

LUPUS *Diary*
Track Your Life with Lupus—
Body, Mind, and Spirit

Gratitude

What am I thankful for today?

_____
_____
_____
_____
_____
_____
_____

More

More thoughts, details, feelings, aha moments about living with Lupus....

_____
_____
_____
_____
_____
_____
_____
_____
_____
_____
_____
_____
_____
_____
_____
_____
_____

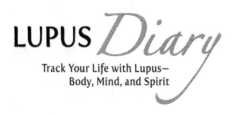

Today's Date:_____

_____

_____

_____

_____

_____

_____

_____

_____

_____

_____

_____

_____

_____

_____

_____

_____

Laughter is inner jogging.

Norman Cousins

Today's Date:_____

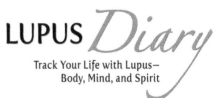

LUPUS *Diary*

Track Your Life with Lupus—
Body, Mind, and Spirit

Body

Today's Habits/Rituals to Soothe My Lupus Body:

○ *Slept Well*　　　　○ *Ate a Clean Diet*　　　○ *Got a Gentle Massage*　　○ *Stayed Hydrated*　　○ *Smiled & Laughed*
○ *Took a Warm Bath*　○ *Moved & Stretched*　○ *Breathed Fresh Air*　　　○ *Protected Skin*　　○ *Was Intimate*

Details and Thoughts About My Physical Symptoms Today:

_____

_____

_____

_____

Mind

Today's Habits/Rituals to Strengthen My Lupus Mind:

○ *Managed Expectations*　○ *Asked for & Accepted Help*　○ *Focused on the Positive*　　○ *Forgave & Released*　○ *Connected*
○ *Managed Time & Energy*　○ *Protected Alone Time*　　　　○ *Managed Stress Response*　○ *Learned About Lupus*　*with My Doctor*

Details and Thoughts About My Emotions Today:

_____

_____

_____

_____

Spirit

Today's Habits/Rituals to Nurture My Lupus Spirit:

○ *Enjoyed Sacred Space*　　　　○ *Cultivated Creativity*　　○ *Embraced Uncertainty*　　○ *Loved Myself*
○ *Meditated, Prayed, Visualized*　○ *Made Someone Happy*　　○ *Worked on Finding and Living My Purpose*

Details and Thoughts About My Spiritual Connection Today:

_____

_____

_____

_____

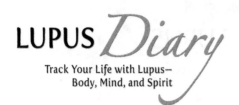 **LUPUS** *Diary*

Track Your Life with Lupus—
Body, Mind, and Spirit

Meals

Breakfast	Lunch	Dinner
_____	_____	_____
_____	_____	_____
_____	_____	_____
_____	_____	_____

Snacks	Water	Reactions to Foods
_____	_____	_____
_____	_____	_____
_____	_____	_____

Notes and Reminders

Items to remember to share with my doctor or other practitioner

_____

_____

_____

_____

_____

_____

_____

_____

_____

_____

Today's Date:_____

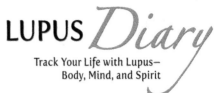
Gratitude

What am I thankful for today?

_____

_____

_____

_____

_____

_____

More

More thoughts, details, feelings, aha moments about living with Lupus....

_____

_____

_____

_____

_____

_____

_____

_____

_____

_____

_____

_____

_____

_____

_____

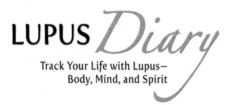

LUPUS *Diary*

Track Your Life with Lupus—
Body, Mind, and Spirit

_____
_____
_____
_____
_____
_____
_____
_____
_____
_____
_____
_____
_____
_____
_____
_____
_____

Start where you are.
Use what you have.
Do what you can.

Arthur Ashe

Today's Date:_____

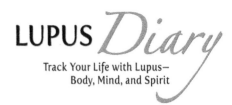

Body

Today's Habits/Rituals to Soothe My Lupus Body:

○ Slept Well   ○ Ate a Clean Diet   ○ Got a Gentle Massage   ○ Stayed Hydrated   ○ Smiled & Laughed

○ Took a Warm Bath   ○ Moved & Stretched   ○ Breathed Fresh Air   ○ Protected Skin   ○ Was Intimate

Details and Thoughts About My Physical Symptoms Today:

_____

_____

_____

_____

Mind

Today's Habits/Rituals to Strengthen My Lupus Mind:

○ Managed Expectations   ○ Asked for & Accepted Help   ○ Focused on the Positive   ○ Forgave & Released   ○ Connected with My Doctor

○ Managed Time & Energy   ○ Protected Alone Time   ○ Managed Stress Response   ○ Learned About Lupus

Details and Thoughts About My Emotions Today:

_____

_____

_____

_____

Spirit

Today's Habits/Rituals to Nurture My Lupus Spirit:

○ Enjoyed Sacred Space   ○ Cultivated Creativity   ○ Embraced Uncertainty   ○ Loved Myself

○ Meditated, Prayed, Visualized   ○ Made Someone Happy   ○ Worked on Finding and Living My Purpose

Details and Thoughts About My Spiritual Connection Today:

_____

_____

_____

_____

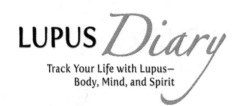

LUPUS *Diary*

Track Your Life with Lupus—
Body, Mind, and Spirit

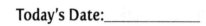

Today's Date:_____

Meals

Breakfast

_____
_____
_____
_____

Lunch

_____
_____
_____
_____

Dinner

_____
_____
_____
_____

Snacks

_____
_____
_____
_____

Water

_____
_____
_____
_____

Reactions to Foods

_____
_____
_____
_____

Notes and Reminders

Items to remember to share with my doctor or other practitioner

_____
_____
_____
_____
_____
_____
_____
_____
_____
_____
_____

Today's Date:_____

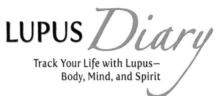

LUPUS *Diary*

Track Your Life with Lupus—
Body, Mind, and Spirit

Gratitude

What am I thankful for today?

_____

_____

_____

_____

_____

_____

_____

More

More thoughts, details, feelings, aha moments about living with Lupus....

_____

_____

_____

_____

_____

_____

_____

_____

_____

_____

_____

_____

_____

_____

_____

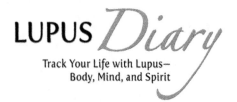

LUPUS *Diary*

Track Your Life with Lupus—
Body, Mind, and Spirit

Today's Date:_____

_____

_____

_____

_____

_____

_____

_____

_____

_____

_____

_____

_____

_____

_____

_____

_____

*Challenges are what make life
interesting and overcoming them
is what makes life meaningful.*

Joshua J. Marine

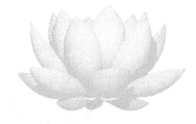

Today's Date:_____

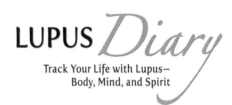

LUPUS *Diary*
Track Your Life with Lupus—
Body, Mind, and Spirit

Body

Today's Habits/Rituals to Soothe My Lupus Body:

○ *Slept Well*　　　○ *Ate a Clean Diet*　　　○ *Got a Gentle Massage*　　　○ *Stayed Hydrated*　　　○ *Smiled & Laughed*
○ *Took a Warm Bath*　　　○ *Moved & Stretched*　　　○ *Breathed Fresh Air*　　　○ *Protected Skin*　　　○ *Was Intimate*

Details and Thoughts About My Physical Symptoms Today:

_____

_____

_____

_____

Mind

Today's Habits/Rituals to Strengthen My Lupus Mind:

○ *Managed Expectations*　　　○ *Asked for & Accepted Help*　　○ *Focused on the Positive*　　　○ *Forgave & Released*　　　○ *Connected with My Doctor*
○ *Managed Time & Energy*　　○ *Protected Alone Time*　　　○ *Managed Stress Response*　　○ *Learned About Lupus*

Details and Thoughts About My Emotions Today:

_____

_____

_____

_____

Spirit

Today's Habits/Rituals to Nurture My Lupus Spirit:

○ *Enjoyed Sacred Space*　　　○ *Cultivated Creativity*　　　○ *Embraced Uncertainty*　　　○ *Loved Myself*
○ *Meditated, Prayed, Visualized*　　　○ *Made Someone Happy*　　　○ *Worked on Finding and Living My Purpose*

Details and Thoughts About My Spiritual Connection Today:

_____

_____

_____

_____

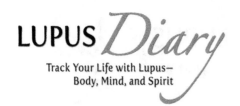 **LUPUS** *Diary*

Track Your Life with Lupus—
Body, Mind, and Spirit

Meals

Breakfast	Lunch	Dinner
_____	_____	_____
_____	_____	_____
_____	_____	_____
_____	_____	_____

Snacks	Water	Reactions to Foods
_____	_____	_____
_____	_____	_____
_____	_____	_____
_____	_____	_____

Notes and Reminders

Items to remember to share with my doctor or other practitioner

_____

_____

_____

_____

_____

_____

_____

_____

_____

_____

_____

Today's Date:_____

Gratitude

What am I thankful for today?

_____

_____

_____

_____

_____

_____

_____

More

More thoughts, details, feelings, aha moments about living with Lupus....

_____

_____

_____

_____

_____

_____

_____

_____

_____

_____

_____

_____

_____

_____

LUPUS *Diary*

Track Your Life with Lupus—
Body, Mind, and Spirit

_____
_____
_____
_____
_____
_____
_____
_____
_____
_____
_____
_____
_____
_____
_____
_____

Writing is a very focused form of meditation. Just as good as sitting in a lotus position.

Alan Moore

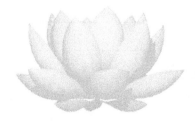

Today's Date:_____

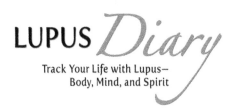

LUPUS *Diary*

Track Your Life with Lupus—
Body, Mind, and Spirit

Body

Today's Habits/Rituals to Soothe My Lupus Body:

○ *Slept Well*   ○ *Ate a Clean Diet*   ○ *Got a Gentle Massage*   ○ *Stayed Hydrated*   ○ *Smiled & Laughed*
○ *Took a Warm Bath*   ○ *Moved & Stretched*   ○ *Breathed Fresh Air*   ○ *Protected Skin*   ○ *Was Intimate*

Details and Thoughts About My Physical Symptoms Today:

_____

_____

_____

_____

Mind

Today's Habits/Rituals to Strengthen My Lupus Mind:

○ *Managed Expectations*   ○ *Asked for & Accepted Help* ○ *Focused on the Positive*   ○ *Forgave & Released*   ○ *Connected*
○ *Managed Time & Energy* ○ *Protected Alone Time*   ○ *Managed Stress Response*   ○ *Learned About Lupus* *with My Doctor*

Details and Thoughts About My Emotions Today:

_____

_____

_____

_____

Spirit

Today's Habits/Rituals to Nurture My Lupus Spirit:

○ *Enjoyed Sacred Space*   ○ *Cultivated Creativity*   ○ *Embraced Uncertainty*   ○ *Loved Myself*
○ *Meditated, Prayed, Visualized* ○ *Made Someone Happy*   ○ *Worked on Finding and Living My Purpose*

Details and Thoughts About My Spiritual Connection Today:

_____

_____

_____

_____

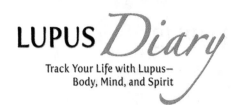**LUPUS** *Diary*

Track Your Life with Lupus—
Body, Mind, and Spirit

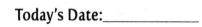**Today's Date:**_____

Meals

Breakfast
_____
_____
_____
_____

Lunch
_____
_____
_____
_____

Dinner
_____
_____
_____
_____

Snacks
_____
_____
_____

Water
_____
_____
_____

Reactions to Foods
_____
_____
_____

Notes and Reminders

Items to remember to share with my doctor or other practitioner
_____
_____
_____
_____
_____
_____
_____
_____
_____
_____
_____

Today's Date:_____

Gratitude

What am I thankful for today?

_____
_____
_____
_____
_____
_____
_____

More

More thoughts, details, feelings, aha moments about living with Lupus....

_____
_____
_____
_____
_____
_____
_____
_____
_____
_____
_____
_____
_____
_____
_____

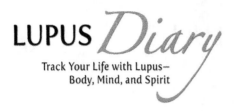

LUPUS *Diary*

Track Your Life with Lupus—
Body, Mind, and Spirit

_____

_____

_____

_____

_____

_____

_____

_____

_____

_____

_____

_____

_____

_____

_____

_____

_____

Don't forget to love yourself.

Soren Kierkegaard

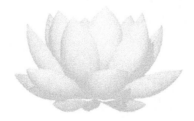

Today's Date:_____

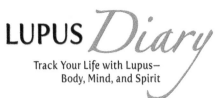

LUPUS *Diary*
Track Your Life with Lupus—
Body, Mind, and Spirit

Body

Today's Habits/Rituals to Soothe My Lupus Body:

○ Slept Well   ○ Ate a Clean Diet   ○ Got a Gentle Massage   ○ Stayed Hydrated   ○ Smiled & Laughed
○ Took a Warm Bath   ○ Moved & Stretched   ○ Breathed Fresh Air   ○ Protected Skin   ○ Was Intimate

Details and Thoughts About My Physical Symptoms Today:

_____

_____

_____

_____

Mind

Today's Habits/Rituals to Strengthen My Lupus Mind:

○ Managed Expectations   ○ Asked for & Accepted Help   ○ Focused on the Positive   ○ Forgave & Released   ○ Connected
○ Managed Time & Energy ○ Protected Alone Time   ○ Managed Stress Response ○ Learned About Lupus   with My
                                                                                                          Doctor

Details and Thoughts About My Emotions Today:

_____

_____

_____

_____

Spirit

Today's Habits/Rituals to Nurture My Lupus Spirit:

○ Enjoyed Sacred Space   ○ Cultivated Creativity   ○ Embraced Uncertainty   ○ Loved Myself
○ Meditated, Prayed, Visualized ○ Made Someone Happy   ○ Worked on Finding and Living My Purpose

Details and Thoughts About My Spiritual Connection Today:

_____

_____

_____

_____

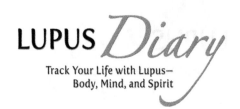
LUPUS *Diary*

Track Your Life with Lupus—
Body, Mind, and Spirit

Meals

Breakfast	Lunch	Dinner
_____	_____	_____
_____	_____	_____
_____	_____	_____
_____	_____	_____

Snacks	Water	Reactions to Foods
_____	_____	_____
_____	_____	_____
_____	_____	_____

Notes and Reminders

Items to remember to share with my doctor or other practitioner

_____

_____

_____

_____

_____

_____

_____

_____

_____

_____

_____

Today's Date:_____

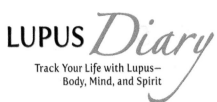

LUPUS *Diary*

Track Your Life with Lupus—
Body, Mind, and Spirit

Gratitude

What am I thankful for today?

_____

_____

_____

_____

_____

_____

More

More thoughts, details, feelings, aha moments about living with Lupus....

_____

_____

_____

_____

_____

_____

_____

_____

_____

_____

_____

_____

_____

_____

_____

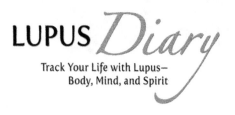
LUPUS *Diary*
Track Your Life with Lupus—
Body, Mind, and Spirit

_____
_____
_____
_____
_____
_____
_____
_____
_____
_____
_____
_____
_____
_____
_____
_____

We shall draw from the heart of suffering itself the means of inspiration and survival.

Winston Churchill

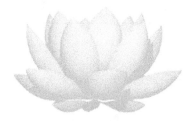

Today's Date:_____

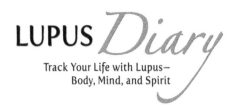

Body

Today's Habits/Rituals to Soothe My Lupus Body:

○ Slept Well ○ Ate a Clean Diet ○ Got a Gentle Massage ○ Stayed Hydrated ○ Smiled & Laughed

○ Took a Warm Bath ○ Moved & Stretched ○ Breathed Fresh Air ○ Protected Skin ○ Was Intimate

Details and Thoughts About My Physical Symptoms Today:

_____

_____

_____

_____

Mind

Today's Habits/Rituals to Strengthen My Lupus Mind:

○ Managed Expectations ○ Asked for & Accepted Help ○ Focused on the Positive ○ Forgave & Released ○ Connected with My Doctor

○ Managed Time & Energy ○ Protected Alone Time ○ Managed Stress Response ○ Learned About Lupus

Details and Thoughts About My Emotions Today:

_____

_____

_____

_____

Spirit

Today's Habits/Rituals to Nurture My Lupus Spirit:

○ Enjoyed Sacred Space ○ Cultivated Creativity ○ Embraced Uncertainty ○ Loved Myself

○ Meditated, Prayed, Visualized ○ Made Someone Happy ○ Worked on Finding and Living My Purpose

Details and Thoughts About My Spiritual Connection Today:

_____

_____

_____

_____

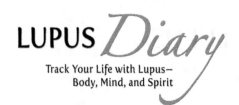

Meals

Breakfast	Lunch	Dinner
_____	_____	_____
_____	_____	_____
_____	_____	_____
_____	_____	_____

Snacks	Water	Reactions to Foods
_____	_____	_____
_____	_____	_____
_____	_____	_____
_____	_____	_____

Notes and Reminders

Items to remember to share with my doctor or other practitioner

_____

_____

_____

_____

_____

_____

_____

_____

_____

_____

_____

Today's Date:_____

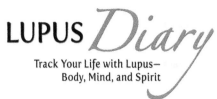
Gratitude

What am I thankful for today?

_____

_____

_____

_____

_____

_____

_____

More

More thoughts, details, feelings, aha moments about living with Lupus....

_____

_____

_____

_____

_____

_____

_____

_____

_____

_____

_____

_____

_____

_____

_____

LUPUS *Diary*

Track Your Life with Lupus—
Body, Mind, and Spirit

_____

_____

_____

_____

_____

_____

_____

_____

_____

_____

_____

_____

_____

_____

_____

_____

_____

Nothing is so healing as the human touch.

Bobby Fischer

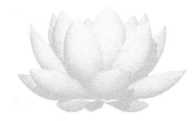

Today's Date:_____

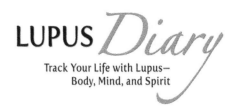

LUPUS *Diary*
Track Your Life with Lupus—
Body, Mind, and Spirit

Body

Today's Habits/Rituals to Soothe My Lupus Body:

○ *Slept Well*   ○ *Ate a Clean Diet*   ○ *Got a Gentle Massage*   ○ *Stayed Hydrated*   ○ *Smiled & Laughed*

○ *Took a Warm Bath*   ○ *Moved & Stretched*   ○ *Breathed Fresh Air*   ○ *Protected Skin*   ○ *Was Intimate*

Details and Thoughts About My Physical Symptoms Today:

_____

_____

_____

_____

Mind

Today's Habits/Rituals to Strengthen My Lupus Mind:

○ *Managed Expectations*   ○ *Asked for & Accepted Help*   ○ *Focused on the Positive*   ○ *Forgave & Released*   ○ *Connected*

○ *Managed Time & Energy*   ○ *Protected Alone Time*   ○ *Managed Stress Response*   ○ *Learned About Lupus*   *with My Doctor*

Details and Thoughts About My Emotions Today:

_____

_____

_____

_____

Spirit

Today's Habits/Rituals to Nurture My Lupus Spirit:

○ *Enjoyed Sacred Space*   ○ *Cultivated Creativity*   ○ *Embraced Uncertainty*   ○ *Loved Myself*

○ *Meditated, Prayed, Visualized*   ○ *Made Someone Happy*   ○ *Worked on Finding and Living My Purpose*

Details and Thoughts About My Spiritual Connection Today:

_____

_____

_____

_____

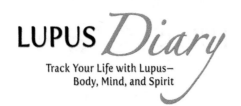 # LUPUS *Diary*

Track Your Life with Lupus—
Body, Mind, and Spirit

Meals

Breakfast	Lunch	Dinner
_____	_____	_____
_____	_____	_____
_____	_____	_____
_____	_____	_____

Snacks	Water	Reactions to Foods
_____	_____	_____
_____	_____	_____
_____	_____	_____

Notes and Reminders

Items to remember to share with my doctor or other practitioner

_____
_____
_____
_____
_____
_____
_____
_____
_____
_____
_____

Today's Date:_____

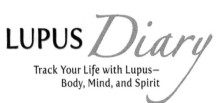

Gratitude

What am I thankful for today?

_____

_____

_____

_____

_____

_____

_____

More

More thoughts, details, feelings, aha moments about living with Lupus....

_____

_____

_____

_____

_____

_____

_____

_____

_____

_____

_____

_____

_____

_____

_____

_____

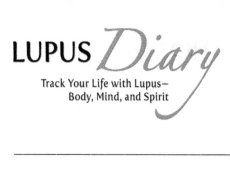

LUPUS *Diary*

Track Your Life with Lupus—
Body, Mind, and Spirit

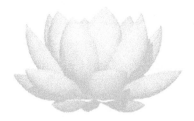

Today's Date:_____

_____
_____
_____
_____
_____
_____
_____
_____
_____
_____
_____
_____
_____
_____
_____
_____

*Movement is a medicine
for creating change in a person's
physical, emotional, and mental states.*

Carol Welch

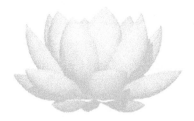

Today's Date:_____

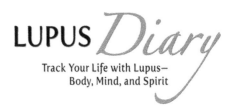

LUPUS *Diary*

Track Your Life with Lupus—
Body, Mind, and Spirit

Body

Today's Habits/Rituals to Soothe My Lupus Body:

○ *Slept Well*   ○ *Ate a Clean Diet*   ○ *Got a Gentle Massage*   ○ *Stayed Hydrated*   ○ *Smiled & Laughed*

○ *Took a Warm Bath*   ○ *Moved & Stretched*   ○ *Breathed Fresh Air*   ○ *Protected Skin*   ○ *Was Intimate*

Details and Thoughts About My Physical Symptoms Today:

_____

_____

_____

_____

Mind

Today's Habits/Rituals to Strengthen My Lupus Mind:

○ *Managed Expectations*   ○ *Asked for & Accepted Help*   ○ *Focused on the Positive*   ○ *Forgave & Released*   ○ *Connected*

○ *Managed Time & Energy*   ○ *Protected Alone Time*   ○ *Managed Stress Response*   ○ *Learned About Lupus*   *with My Doctor*

Details and Thoughts About My Emotions Today:

_____

_____

_____

_____

Spirit

Today's Habits/Rituals to Nurture My Lupus Spirit:

○ *Enjoyed Sacred Space*   ○ *Cultivated Creativity*   ○ *Embraced Uncertainty*   ○ *Loved Myself*

○ *Meditated, Prayed, Visualized*   ○ *Made Someone Happy*   ○ *Worked on Finding and Living My Purpose*

Details and Thoughts About My Spiritual Connection Today:

_____

_____

_____

_____

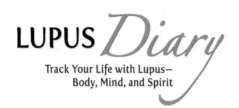 **LUPUS** *Diary*

Track Your Life with Lupus—
Body, Mind, and Spirit

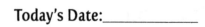 **Today's Date:**_____

Meals

Breakfast	Lunch	Dinner
_____	_____	_____
_____	_____	_____
_____	_____	_____
_____	_____	_____

Snacks	Water	Reactions to Foods
_____	_____	_____
_____	_____	_____
_____	_____	_____
_____	_____	_____

Notes and Reminders

Items to remember to share with my doctor or other practitioner

_____
_____
_____
_____
_____
_____
_____
_____
_____
_____
_____

Today's Date:_____

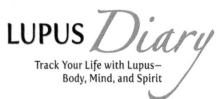

Gratitude

What am I thankful for today?

_____

_____

_____

_____

_____

_____

_____

More

More thoughts, details, feelings, aha moments about living with Lupus....

_____

_____

_____

_____

_____

_____

_____

_____

_____

_____

_____

_____

_____

_____

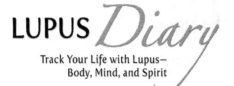

LUPUS *Diary*

Track Your Life with Lupus—
Body, Mind, and Spirit

_____

_____

_____

_____

_____

_____

_____

_____

_____

_____

_____

_____

_____

_____

_____

_____

_____

_____

*Fresh air impoverishes
the doctor.*

Danish Proverb

Today's Date:_____

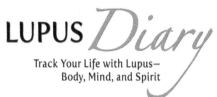
LUPUS *Diary*
Track Your Life with Lupus—
Body, Mind, and Spirit

Body

Today's Habits/Rituals to Soothe My Lupus Body:

○ *Slept Well*　　　○ *Ate a Clean Diet*　　　○ *Got a Gentle Massage*　　　○ *Stayed Hydrated*　　　○ *Smiled & Laughed*

○ *Took a Warm Bath*　　○ *Moved & Stretched*　　○ *Breathed Fresh Air*　　○ *Protected Skin*　　○ *Was Intimate*

Details and Thoughts About My Physical Symptoms Today:

_____

_____

_____

_____

Mind

Today's Habits/Rituals to Strengthen My Lupus Mind:

○ *Managed Expectations*　○ *Asked for & Accepted Help*　○ *Focused on the Positive*　○ *Forgave & Released*　○ *Connected with My Doctor*

○ *Managed Time & Energy*　○ *Protected Alone Time*　　○ *Managed Stress Response*　○ *Learned About Lupus*

Details and Thoughts About My Emotions Today:

_____

_____

_____

_____

Spirit

Today's Habits/Rituals to Nurture My Lupus Spirit:

○ *Enjoyed Sacred Space*　　　○ *Cultivated Creativity*　　○ *Embraced Uncertainty*　　○ *Loved Myself*

○ *Meditated, Prayed, Visualized*　○ *Made Someone Happy*　○ *Worked on Finding and Living My Purpose*

Details and Thoughts About My Spiritual Connection Today:

_____

_____

_____

_____

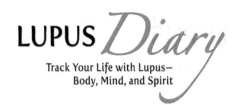

LUPUS *Diary*

Track Your Life with Lupus—
Body, Mind, and Spirit

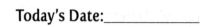

Today's Date:_____

Meals

Breakfast	Lunch	Dinner
_____	_____	_____
_____	_____	_____
_____	_____	_____
_____	_____	_____

Snacks	Water	Reactions to Foods
_____	_____	_____
_____	_____	_____
_____	_____	_____
_____	_____	_____

Notes and Reminders

Items to remember to share with my doctor or other practitioner

_____

_____

_____

_____

_____

_____

_____

_____

_____

_____

Today's Date:_____

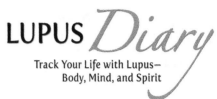

LUPUS *Diary*

Track Your Life with Lupus—
Body, Mind, and Spirit

Gratitude

What am I thankful for today?

_____
_____
_____
_____
_____
_____
_____

More

More thoughts, details, feelings, aha moments about living with Lupus....

_____
_____
_____
_____
_____
_____
_____
_____
_____
_____
_____
_____
_____
_____
_____
_____

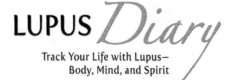

LUPUS *Diary*

Track Your Life with Lupus—
Body, Mind, and Spirit

Today's Date:_____

_____
_____
_____
_____
_____
_____
_____
_____
_____
_____
_____
_____
_____
_____
_____
_____

The quieter you become,
the more you can hear.

Baba Ram Dass

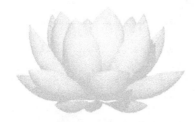

Today's Date:_____

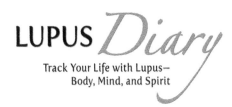

LUPUS *Diary*

Track Your Life with Lupus—
Body, Mind, and Spirit

Body

Today's Habits/Rituals to Soothe My Lupus Body:

○ *Slept Well*   ○ *Ate a Clean Diet*   ○ *Got a Gentle Massage*   ○ *Stayed Hydrated*   ○ *Smiled & Laughed*

○ *Took a Warm Bath*   ○ *Moved & Stretched*   ○ *Breathed Fresh Air*   ○ *Protected Skin*   ○ *Was Intimate*

Details and Thoughts About My Physical Symptoms Today:

_____

_____

_____

_____

Mind

Today's Habits/Rituals to Strengthen My Lupus Mind:

○ *Managed Expectations*   ○ *Asked for & Accepted Help*   ○ *Focused on the Positive*   ○ *Forgave & Released*   ○ *Connected with My Doctor*

○ *Managed Time & Energy*   ○ *Protected Alone Time*   ○ *Managed Stress Response*   ○ *Learned About Lupus*

Details and Thoughts About My Emotions Today:

_____

_____

_____

_____

Spirit

Today's Habits/Rituals to Nurture My Lupus Spirit:

○ *Enjoyed Sacred Space*   ○ *Cultivated Creativity*   ○ *Embraced Uncertainty*   ○ *Loved Myself*

○ *Meditated, Prayed, Visualized*   ○ *Made Someone Happy*   ○ *Worked on Finding and Living My Purpose*

Details and Thoughts About My Spiritual Connection Today:

_____

_____

_____

_____

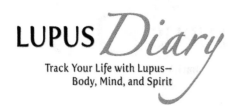 **LUPUS** *Diary*

Track Your Life with Lupus—
Body, Mind, and Spirit

 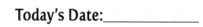

Meals

Breakfast

_____
_____
_____
_____

Lunch

_____
_____
_____
_____

Dinner

_____
_____
_____
_____

Snacks

_____
_____
_____
_____

Water

_____
_____
_____
_____

Reactions to Foods

_____
_____
_____
_____

Notes and Reminders

Items to remember to share with my doctor or other practitioner

_____
_____
_____
_____
_____
_____
_____
_____
_____
_____

Today's Date:_____

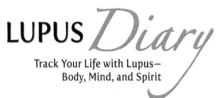

LUPUS *Diary*

Track Your Life with Lupus—
Body, Mind, and Spirit

Gratitude

What am I thankful for today?

_____

_____

_____

_____

_____

_____

More

More thoughts, details, feelings, aha moments about living with Lupus....

_____

_____

_____

_____

_____

_____

_____

_____

_____

_____

_____

_____

_____

_____

_____

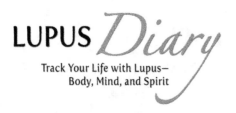

LUPUS *Diary*

Track Your Life with Lupus—
Body, Mind, and Spirit

<inline>Today's Date:_____</inline>

_____
_____
_____
_____
_____
_____
_____
_____
_____
_____
_____
_____
_____
_____
_____
_____
_____

*Acceptance doesn't mean resignation; it means
understanding that something is what it is
and that there's got to be a way through it.*

Michael J. Fox

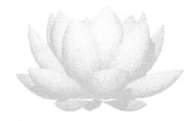

Today's Date:_____

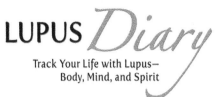

LUPUS *Diary*

Track Your Life with Lupus—
Body, Mind, and Spirit

Body

Today's Habits/Rituals to Soothe My Lupus Body:

○ *Slept Well*　　　○ *Ate a Clean Diet*　　　○ *Got a Gentle Massage*　　　○ *Stayed Hydrated*　　　○ *Smiled & Laughed*

○ *Took a Warm Bath*　　○ *Moved & Stretched*　　○ *Breathed Fresh Air*　　○ *Protected Skin*　　○ *Was Intimate*

Details and Thoughts About My Physical Symptoms Today:

_____

_____

_____

_____

Mind

Today's Habits/Rituals to Strengthen My Lupus Mind:

○ *Managed Expectations*　○ *Asked for & Accepted Help*　○ *Focused on the Positive*　○ *Forgave & Released*　○ *Connected with My Doctor*

○ *Managed Time & Energy*　○ *Protected Alone Time*　　○ *Managed Stress Response*　○ *Learned About Lupus*

Details and Thoughts About My Emotions Today:

_____

_____

_____

_____

Spirit

Today's Habits/Rituals to Nurture My Lupus Spirit:

○ *Enjoyed Sacred Space*　　　○ *Cultivated Creativity*　　　○ *Embraced Uncertainty*　　　○ *Loved Myself*

○ *Meditated, Prayed, Visualized*　　○ *Made Someone Happy*　　○ *Worked on Finding and Living My Purpose*

Details and Thoughts About My Spiritual Connection Today:

_____

_____

_____

_____

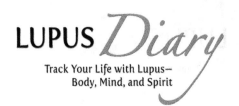

LUPUS *Diary*
Track Your Life with Lupus—
Body, Mind, and Spirit

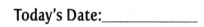

Today's Date:_____

Meals

Breakfast

_____

_____

_____

_____

Lunch

_____

_____

_____

_____

Dinner

_____

_____

_____

_____

Snacks

_____

_____

_____

_____

Water

_____

_____

_____

_____

Reactions to Foods

_____

_____

_____

_____

Notes and Reminders

Items to remember to share with my doctor or other practitioner

_____

_____

_____

_____

_____

_____

_____

_____

_____

_____

_____

Today's Date:_____

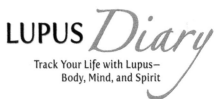

Gratitude

What am I thankful for today?

_____

_____

_____

_____

_____

_____

_____

More

More thoughts, details, feelings, aha moments about living with Lupus....

_____

_____

_____

_____

_____

_____

_____

_____

_____

_____

_____

_____

_____

_____

_____

_____

_____

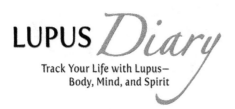

LUPUS *Diary*

Track Your Life with Lupus—
Body, Mind, and Spirit

Today's Date:_____

_____
_____
_____
_____
_____
_____
_____
_____
_____
_____
_____
_____
_____
_____
_____
_____
_____

It's not stress that kills us,
it is our reaction to it.

Hans Selye

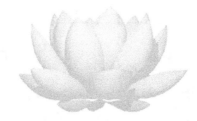

Today's Date:_____

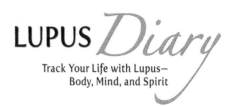

LUPUS *Diary*

Track Your Life with Lupus—
Body, Mind, and Spirit

Body

Today's Habits/Rituals to Soothe My Lupus Body:

○ Slept Well   ○ Ate a Clean Diet   ○ Got a Gentle Massage   ○ Stayed Hydrated   ○ Smiled & Laughed

○ Took a Warm Bath   ○ Moved & Stretched   ○ Breathed Fresh Air   ○ Protected Skin   ○ Was Intimate

Details and Thoughts About My Physical Symptoms Today:

_____

_____

_____

_____

Mind

Today's Habits/Rituals to Strengthen My Lupus Mind:

○ Managed Expectations   ○ Asked for & Accepted Help   ○ Focused on the Positive   ○ Forgave & Released   ○ Connected

○ Managed Time & Energy ○ Protected Alone Time   ○ Managed Stress Response   ○ Learned About Lupus   with My Doctor

Details and Thoughts About My Emotions Today:

_____

_____

_____

_____

Spirit

Today's Habits/Rituals to Nurture My Lupus Spirit:

○ Enjoyed Sacred Space   ○ Cultivated Creativity   ○ Embraced Uncertainty   ○ Loved Myself

○ Meditated, Prayed, Visualized ○ Made Someone Happy   ○ Worked on Finding and Living My Purpose

Details and Thoughts About My Spiritual Connection Today:

_____

_____

_____

_____

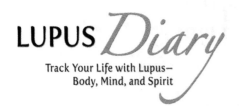 **LUPUS** *Diary*

Track Your Life with Lupus—
Body, Mind, and Spirit

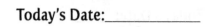 **Today's Date:**_____

Meals

Breakfast

_____

_____

_____

_____

Lunch

_____

_____

_____

_____

Dinner

_____

_____

_____

_____

Snacks

_____

_____

_____

Water

_____

_____

_____

Reactions to Foods

_____

_____

_____

Notes and Reminders

Items to remember to share with my doctor or other practitioner

_____

_____

_____

_____

_____

_____

_____

_____

_____

_____

_____

Today's Date: _____

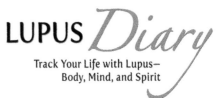

LUPUS *Diary*
Track Your Life with Lupus—
Body, Mind, and Spirit

Gratitude

What am I thankful for today?

_____

_____

_____

_____

_____

_____

More

More thoughts, details, feelings, aha moments about living with Lupus....

_____

_____

_____

_____

_____

_____

_____

_____

_____

_____

_____

_____

_____

_____

_____

_____

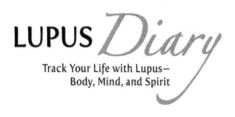

LUPUS *Diary*

Track Your Life with Lupus—
Body, Mind, and Spirit

Today's Date:_____

_____

_____

_____

_____

_____

_____

_____

_____

_____

_____

_____

_____

_____

_____

_____

_____

Fall seven times and stand up eight.

Japanese Proverb

Today's Date:_____

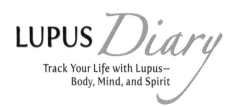

LUPUS *Diary*
Track Your Life with Lupus—
Body, Mind, and Spirit

Body

Today's Habits/Rituals to Soothe My Lupus Body:

○ *Slept Well*   ○ *Ate a Clean Diet*   ○ *Got a Gentle Massage*   ○ *Stayed Hydrated*   ○ *Smiled & Laughed*

○ *Took a Warm Bath*   ○ *Moved & Stretched*   ○ *Breathed Fresh Air*   ○ *Protected Skin*   ○ *Was Intimate*

Details and Thoughts About My Physical Symptoms Today:

_____

_____

_____

_____

Mind

Today's Habits/Rituals to Strengthen My Lupus Mind:

○ *Managed Expectations*   ○ *Asked for & Accepted Help*   ○ *Focused on the Positive*   ○ *Forgave & Released*   ○ *Connected with My Doctor*

○ *Managed Time & Energy*   ○ *Protected Alone Time*   ○ *Managed Stress Response*   ○ *Learned About Lupus*

Details and Thoughts About My Emotions Today:

_____

_____

_____

_____

Spirit

Today's Habits/Rituals to Nurture My Lupus Spirit:

○ *Enjoyed Sacred Space*   ○ *Cultivated Creativity*   ○ *Embraced Uncertainty*   ○ *Loved Myself*

○ *Meditated, Prayed, Visualized*   ○ *Made Someone Happy*   ○ *Worked on Finding and Living My Purpose*

Details and Thoughts About My Spiritual Connection Today:

_____

_____

_____

_____

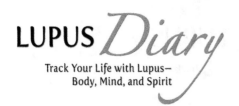**LUPUS** *Diary*

Track Your Life with Lupus—
Body, Mind, and Spirit

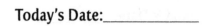

Meals

Breakfast

_____
_____
_____
_____

Lunch

_____
_____
_____
_____

Dinner

_____
_____
_____
_____

Snacks

_____
_____
_____

Water

_____
_____
_____

Reactions to Foods

_____
_____
_____

Notes and Reminders

Items to remember to share with my doctor or other practitioner

_____
_____
_____
_____
_____
_____
_____
_____
_____
_____
_____

Today's Date:_____

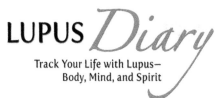

LUPUS *Diary*
Track Your Life with Lupus—
Body, Mind, and Spirit

Gratitude

What am I thankful for today?

_____

_____

_____

_____

_____

_____

_____

More

More thoughts, details, feelings, aha moments about living with Lupus....

_____

_____

_____

_____

_____

_____

_____

_____

_____

_____

_____

_____

_____

_____

_____

_____

_____

_____

_____

_____

_____

_____

_____

_____

_____

_____

_____

_____

_____

_____

_____

_____

*It is during our darkest moments
that we must focus
to see the light.*

Aristotle Onassis

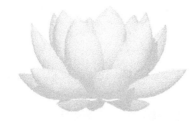

Today's Date:_____

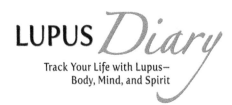

Body

Today's Habits/Rituals to Soothe My Lupus Body:

○ Slept Well   ○ Ate a Clean Diet   ○ Got a Gentle Massage   ○ Stayed Hydrated   ○ Smiled & Laughed

○ Took a Warm Bath   ○ Moved & Stretched   ○ Breathed Fresh Air   ○ Protected Skin   ○ Was Intimate

Details and Thoughts About My Physical Symptoms Today:

_____

_____

_____

_____

Mind

Today's Habits/Rituals to Strengthen My Lupus Mind:

○ Managed Expectations ○ Asked for & Accepted Help ○ Focused on the Positive ○ Forgave & Released ○ Connected with My Doctor

○ Managed Time & Energy ○ Protected Alone Time ○ Managed Stress Response ○ Learned About Lupus

Details and Thoughts About My Emotions Today:

_____

_____

_____

_____

Spirit

Today's Habits/Rituals to Nurture My Lupus Spirit:

○ Enjoyed Sacred Space   ○ Cultivated Creativity   ○ Embraced Uncertainty   ○ Loved Myself

○ Meditated, Prayed, Visualized   ○ Made Someone Happy   ○ Worked on Finding and Living My Purpose

Details and Thoughts About My Spiritual Connection Today:

_____

_____

_____

_____

LUPUS *Diary*

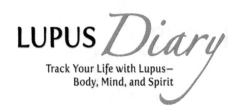

Track Your Life with Lupus—
Body, Mind, and Spirit

Meals

Breakfast

_____

_____

_____

_____

Lunch

_____

_____

_____

_____

Dinner

_____

_____

_____

_____

Snacks

_____

_____

_____

Water

_____

_____

_____

Reactions to Foods

_____

_____

_____

Notes and Reminders

Items to remember to share with my doctor or other practitioner

_____

_____

_____

_____

_____

_____

_____

_____

_____

_____

_____

Today's Date:_____

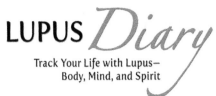

Gratitude

What am I thankful for today?

_____

_____

_____

_____

_____

_____

_____

More

More thoughts, details, feelings, aha moments about living with Lupus....

_____

_____

_____

_____

_____

_____

_____

_____

_____

_____

_____

_____

_____

_____

_____

_____

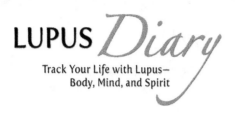

LUPUS *Diary*

Track Your Life with Lupus—
Body, Mind, and Spirit

Today's Date:_____

_____

_____

_____

_____

_____

_____

_____

_____

_____

_____

_____

_____

_____

_____

_____

_____

_____

Be still and cool
in thine own mind and spirit.

George Fox

Today's Date:_____

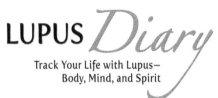

LUPUS *Diary*

Track Your Life with Lupus—
Body, Mind, and Spirit

Body

Today's Habits/Rituals to Soothe My Lupus Body:

○ Slept Well ○ Ate a Clean Diet ○ Got a Gentle Massage ○ Stayed Hydrated ○ Smiled & Laughed
○ Took a Warm Bath ○ Moved & Stretched ○ Breathed Fresh Air ○ Protected Skin ○ Was Intimate

Details and Thoughts About My Physical Symptoms Today:

_____

_____

_____

_____

Mind

Today's Habits/Rituals to Strengthen My Lupus Mind:

○ Managed Expectations ○ Asked for & Accepted Help ○ Focused on the Positive ○ Forgave & Released ○ Connected with My Doctor
○ Managed Time & Energy ○ Protected Alone Time ○ Managed Stress Response ○ Learned About Lupus

Details and Thoughts About My Emotions Today:

_____

_____

_____

_____

Spirit

Today's Habits/Rituals to Nurture My Lupus Spirit:

○ Enjoyed Sacred Space ○ Cultivated Creativity ○ Embraced Uncertainty ○ Loved Myself
○ Meditated, Prayed, Visualized ○ Made Someone Happy ○ Worked on Finding and Living My Purpose

Details and Thoughts About My Spiritual Connection Today:

_____

_____

_____

_____

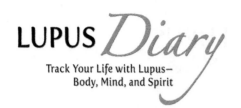 **LUPUS** *Diary*

Track Your Life with Lupus—
Body, Mind, and Spirit

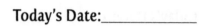

Meals

Breakfast	Lunch	Dinner
_____	_____	_____
_____	_____	_____
_____	_____	_____
_____	_____	_____

Snacks	Water	Reactions to Foods
_____	_____	_____
_____	_____	_____
_____	_____	_____
_____	_____	_____

Notes and Reminders

Items to remember to share with my doctor or other practitioner

_____

_____

_____

_____

_____

_____

_____

_____

_____

_____

Today's Date:_____

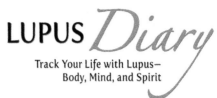

LUPUS *Diary*

Track Your Life with Lupus—
Body, Mind, and Spirit

Gratitude

What am I thankful for today?

_____

_____

_____

_____

_____

_____

More

More thoughts, details, feelings, aha moments about living with Lupus....

_____

_____

_____

_____

_____

_____

_____

_____

_____

_____

_____

_____

_____

_____

_____

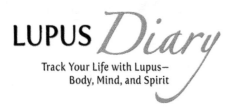

LUPUS *Diary*

Track Your Life with Lupus—
Body, Mind, and Spirit

_____
_____
_____
_____
_____
_____
_____
_____
_____
_____
_____
_____
_____
_____
_____
_____
_____
_____

*A hero is an ordinary individual who finds
the strength to persevere and endure
in spite of overwhelming obstacles.*

Christopher Reeves

Today's Date:_____

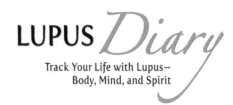

LUPUS *Diary*

Track Your Life with Lupus—
Body, Mind, and Spirit

Body

Today's Habits/Rituals to Soothe My Lupus Body:

○ *Slept Well*　　　○ *Ate a Clean Diet*　　○ *Got a Gentle Massage*　　○ *Stayed Hydrated*　　○ *Smiled & Laughed*

○ *Took a Warm Bath*　○ *Moved & Stretched*　○ *Breathed Fresh Air*　　　○ *Protected Skin*　　○ *Was Intimate*

Details and Thoughts About My Physical Symptoms Today:

_____

_____

_____

_____

Mind

Today's Habits/Rituals to Strengthen My Lupus Mind:

○ *Managed Expectations*　○ *Asked for & Accepted Help*　○ *Focused on the Positive*　○ *Forgave & Released*　○ *Connected with My Doctor*

○ *Managed Time & Energy*　○ *Protected Alone Time*　　　○ *Managed Stress Response*　○ *Learned About Lupus*

Details and Thoughts About My Emotions Today:

_____

_____

_____

_____

Spirit

Today's Habits/Rituals to Nurture My Lupus Spirit:

○ *Enjoyed Sacred Space*　　　○ *Cultivated Creativity*　　○ *Embraced Uncertainty*　　○ *Loved Myself*

○ *Meditated, Prayed, Visualized*　○ *Made Someone Happy*　○ *Worked on Finding and Living My Purpose*

Details and Thoughts About My Spiritual Connection Today:

_____

_____

_____

_____

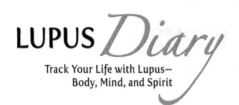
LUPUS *Diary*
Track Your Life with Lupus—
Body, Mind, and Spirit

Meals

Breakfast

_____
_____
_____
_____

Lunch

_____
_____
_____
_____

Dinner

_____
_____
_____
_____

Snacks

_____
_____
_____

Water

_____
_____
_____

Reactions to Foods

_____
_____
_____

Notes and Reminders

Items to remember to share with my doctor or other practitioner

_____
_____
_____
_____
_____
_____
_____
_____
_____
_____
_____

Today's Date:_____

Gratitude

What am I thankful for today?

_____

_____

_____

_____

_____

_____

_____

More

More thoughts, details, feelings, aha moments about living with Lupus....

_____

_____

_____

_____

_____

_____

_____

_____

_____

_____

_____

_____

_____

_____

_____

_____

_____

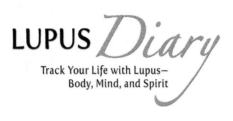
_____

_____

_____

_____

_____

_____

_____

_____

_____

_____

_____

_____

_____

_____

_____

_____

_____

It is through gratitude for the present moment that the spiritual dimension of life opens up.

Eckhart Tolle

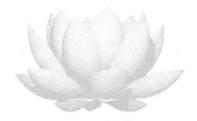

Today's Date:_____

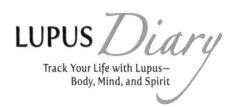

LUPUS *Diary*

Track Your Life with Lupus—
Body, Mind, and Spirit

Body

Today's Habits/Rituals to Soothe My Lupus Body:

○ Slept Well　　　○ Ate a Clean Diet　　　○ Got a Gentle Massage　　　○ Stayed Hydrated　　　○ Smiled & Laughed

○ Took a Warm Bath　　　○ Moved & Stretched　　　○ Breathed Fresh Air　　　○ Protected Skin　　　○ Was Intimate

Details and Thoughts About My Physical Symptoms Today:

_____

_____

_____

_____

Mind

Today's Habits/Rituals to Strengthen My Lupus Mind:

○ Managed Expectations　○ Asked for & Accepted Help　○ Focused on the Positive　○ Forgave & Released　○ Connected with My Doctor

○ Managed Time & Energy　○ Protected Alone Time　　○ Managed Stress Response　○ Learned About Lupus

Details and Thoughts About My Emotions Today:

_____

_____

_____

_____

Spirit

Today's Habits/Rituals to Nurture My Lupus Spirit:

○ Enjoyed Sacred Space　　　○ Cultivated Creativity　　　○ Embraced Uncertainty　　　○ Loved Myself

○ Meditated, Prayed, Visualized　　　○ Made Someone Happy　　　○ Worked on Finding and Living My Purpose

Details and Thoughts About My Spiritual Connection Today:

_____

_____

_____

_____

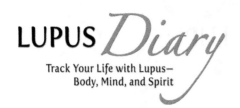

LUPUS *Diary*

Track Your Life with Lupus—
Body, Mind, and Spirit

Today's Date: 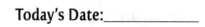_____

Meals

Breakfast	Lunch	Dinner
_____	_____	_____
_____	_____	_____
_____	_____	_____
_____	_____	_____

Snacks	Water	Reactions to Foods
_____	_____	_____
_____	_____	_____
_____	_____	_____

Notes and Reminders

Items to remember to share with my doctor or other practitioner

_____

_____

_____

_____

_____

_____

_____

_____

_____

_____

_____

_____

Today's Date:_____

Gratitude

What am I thankful for today?

_____

_____

_____

_____

_____

_____

_____

More

More thoughts, details, feelings, aha moments about living with Lupus....

_____

_____

_____

_____

_____

_____

_____

_____

_____

_____

_____

_____

_____

_____

_____

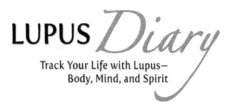

LUPUS *Diary*

Track Your Life with Lupus—
Body, Mind, and Spirit

Today's Date:_____

_____

_____

_____

_____

_____

_____

_____

_____

_____

_____

_____

_____

_____

_____

_____

_____

Trust yourself,
you know more than
you think you do.

Benjamin Spock

Today's Date:_____

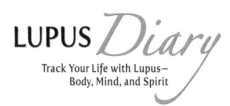

LUPUS *Diary*
Track Your Life with Lupus—
Body, Mind, and Spirit

Body

Today's Habits/Rituals to Soothe My Lupus Body:

○ *Slept Well*   ○ *Ate a Clean Diet*   ○ *Got a Gentle Massage*   ○ *Stayed Hydrated*   ○ *Smiled & Laughed*

○ *Took a Warm Bath*   ○ *Moved & Stretched*   ○ *Breathed Fresh Air*   ○ *Protected Skin*   ○ *Was Intimate*

Details and Thoughts About My Physical Symptoms Today:

_____

_____

_____

_____

Mind

Today's Habits/Rituals to Strengthen My Lupus Mind:

○ *Managed Expectations*   ○ *Asked for & Accepted Help*   ○ *Focused on the Positive*   ○ *Forgave & Released*   ○ *Connected with My Doctor*

○ *Managed Time & Energy*   ○ *Protected Alone Time*   ○ *Managed Stress Response*   ○ *Learned About Lupus*

Details and Thoughts About My Emotions Today:

_____

_____

_____

_____

Spirit

Today's Habits/Rituals to Nurture My Lupus Spirit:

○ *Enjoyed Sacred Space*   ○ *Cultivated Creativity*   ○ *Embraced Uncertainty*   ○ *Loved Myself*

○ *Meditated, Prayed, Visualized*   ○ *Made Someone Happy*   ○ *Worked on Finding and Living My Purpose*

Details and Thoughts About My Spiritual Connection Today:

_____

_____

_____

_____

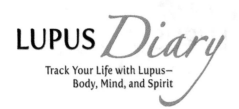

Meals

Breakfast

_____
_____
_____
_____

Lunch

_____
_____
_____
_____

Dinner

_____
_____
_____
_____

Snacks

_____
_____
_____
_____

Water

_____
_____
_____
_____

Reactions to Foods

_____
_____
_____
_____

Notes and Reminders

Items to remember to share with my doctor or other practitioner

_____
_____
_____
_____
_____
_____
_____
_____
_____
_____
_____

Today's Date:_____

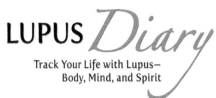

LUPUS *Diary*

Track Your Life with Lupus—
Body, Mind, and Spirit

Gratitude

What am I thankful for today?

_____

_____

_____

_____

_____

_____

_____

More

More thoughts, details, feelings, aha moments about living with Lupus....

_____

_____

_____

_____

_____

_____

_____

_____

_____

_____

_____

_____

_____

_____

_____

LUPUS *Diary*

Track Your Life with Lupus—
Body, Mind, and Spirit

Today's Date:_____

_____

_____

_____

_____

_____

_____

_____

_____

_____

_____

_____

_____

_____

_____

_____

_____

*Man never made any material
as resilient as the human spirit.*

Bernard Williams

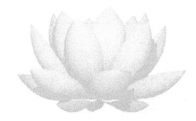

Today's Date:_____

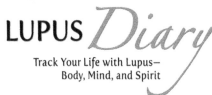

LUPUS *Diary*

Track Your Life with Lupus—
Body, Mind, and Spirit

Body

Today's Habits/Rituals to Soothe My Lupus Body:

○ *Slept Well*   ○ *Ate a Clean Diet*   ○ *Got a Gentle Massage*   ○ *Stayed Hydrated*   ○ *Smiled & Laughed*

○ *Took a Warm Bath*   ○ *Moved & Stretched*   ○ *Breathed Fresh Air*   ○ *Protected Skin*   ○ *Was Intimate*

Details and Thoughts About My Physical Symptoms Today:

_____

_____

_____

_____

Mind

Today's Habits/Rituals to Strengthen My Lupus Mind:

○ *Managed Expectations*   ○ *Asked for & Accepted Help*   ○ *Focused on the Positive*   ○ *Forgave & Released*   ○ *Connected with My Doctor*

○ *Managed Time & Energy*   ○ *Protected Alone Time*   ○ *Managed Stress Response*   ○ *Learned About Lupus*

Details and Thoughts About My Emotions Today:

_____

_____

_____

_____

Spirit

Today's Habits/Rituals to Nurture My Lupus Spirit:

○ *Enjoyed Sacred Space*   ○ *Cultivated Creativity*   ○ *Embraced Uncertainty*   ○ *Loved Myself*

○ *Meditated, Prayed, Visualized*   ○ *Made Someone Happy*   ○ *Worked on Finding and Living My Purpose*

Details and Thoughts About My Spiritual Connection Today:

_____

_____

_____

_____

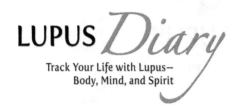
LUPUS *Diary*
Track Your Life with Lupus—
Body, Mind, and Spirit

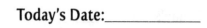
Today's Date:_____

Meals

Breakfast

_____

_____

_____

_____

Lunch

_____

_____

_____

_____

Dinner

_____

_____

_____

_____

Snacks

_____

_____

_____

_____

Water

_____

_____

_____

_____

Reactions to Foods

_____

_____

_____

_____

Notes and Reminders

Items to remember to share with my doctor or other practitioner

_____

_____

_____

_____

_____

_____

_____

_____

_____

_____

_____

Today's Date:_____

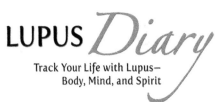

Gratitude

What am I thankful for today?

_____

_____

_____

_____

_____

_____

_____

More

More thoughts, details, feelings, aha moments about living with Lupus....

_____

_____

_____

_____

_____

_____

_____

_____

_____

_____

_____

_____

_____

_____

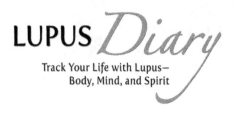
_____

_____

_____

_____

_____

_____

_____

_____

_____

_____

_____

_____

_____

_____

_____

_____

*Faith means living with uncertainty—
feeling your way through life, letting your heart
guide you like a lantern in the dark.*

Dan Millman

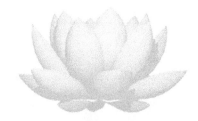

Today's Date:_____

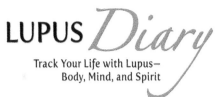

Body

Today's Habits/Rituals to Soothe My Lupus Body:

○ Slept Well   ○ Ate a Clean Diet   ○ Got a Gentle Massage   ○ Stayed Hydrated   ○ Smiled & Laughed

○ Took a Warm Bath   ○ Moved & Stretched   ○ Breathed Fresh Air   ○ Protected Skin   ○ Was Intimate

Details and Thoughts About My Physical Symptoms Today:

_____

_____

_____

_____

Mind

Today's Habits/Rituals to Strengthen My Lupus Mind:

○ Managed Expectations   ○ Asked for & Accepted Help   ○ Focused on the Positive   ○ Forgave & Released   ○ Connected with My Doctor

○ Managed Time & Energy   ○ Protected Alone Time   ○ Managed Stress Response   ○ Learned About Lupus

Details and Thoughts About My Emotions Today:

_____

_____

_____

_____

Spirit

Today's Habits/Rituals to Nurture My Lupus Spirit:

○ Enjoyed Sacred Space   ○ Cultivated Creativity   ○ Embraced Uncertainty   ○ Loved Myself

○ Meditated, Prayed, Visualized   ○ Made Someone Happy   ○ Worked on Finding and Living My Purpose

Details and Thoughts About My Spiritual Connection Today:

_____

_____

_____

_____

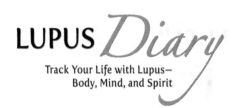

LUPUS *Diary*

Track Your Life with Lupus—
Body, Mind, and Spirit

Today's Date:_____

Meals

Breakfast	Lunch	Dinner
_____	_____	_____
_____	_____	_____
_____	_____	_____
_____	_____	_____

Snacks	Water	Reactions to Foods
_____	_____	_____
_____	_____	_____
_____	_____	_____
_____	_____	_____

Notes and Reminders

Items to remember to share with my doctor or other practitioner

_____

_____

_____

_____

_____

_____

_____

_____

_____

_____

_____

Today's Date:_____

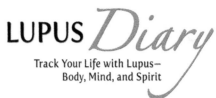

Gratitude

What am I thankful for today?

_____

_____

_____

_____

_____

_____

More

More thoughts, details, feelings, aha moments about living with Lupus....

_____

_____

_____

_____

_____

_____

_____

_____

_____

_____

_____

_____

_____

_____

_____

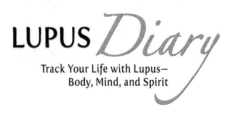

LUPUS *Diary*

Track Your Life with Lupus—
Body, Mind, and Spirit

Today's Date:_____

_____
_____
_____
_____
_____
_____
_____
_____
_____
_____
_____
_____
_____
_____
_____
_____

Forgive and release. Do not allow hurts to burrow within.

Unknown

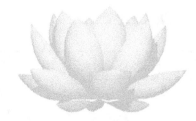

Today's Date:_____

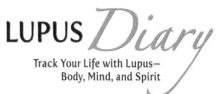

Body

Today's Habits/Rituals to Soothe My Lupus Body:

○ Slept Well   ○ Ate a Clean Diet   ○ Got a Gentle Massage   ○ Stayed Hydrated   ○ Smiled & Laughed

○ Took a Warm Bath   ○ Moved & Stretched   ○ Breathed Fresh Air   ○ Protected Skin   ○ Was Intimate

Details and Thoughts About My Physical Symptoms Today:

_____

_____

_____

_____

Mind

Today's Habits/Rituals to Strengthen My Lupus Mind:

○ Managed Expectations   ○ Asked for & Accepted Help   ○ Focused on the Positive   ○ Forgave & Released   ○ Connected with My Doctor

○ Managed Time & Energy   ○ Protected Alone Time   ○ Managed Stress Response   ○ Learned About Lupus

Details and Thoughts About My Emotions Today:

_____

_____

_____

_____

Spirit

Today's Habits/Rituals to Nurture My Lupus Spirit:

○ Enjoyed Sacred Space   ○ Cultivated Creativity   ○ Embraced Uncertainty   ○ Loved Myself

○ Meditated, Prayed, Visualized   ○ Made Someone Happy   ○ Worked on Finding and Living My Purpose

Details and Thoughts About My Spiritual Connection Today:

_____

_____

_____

_____

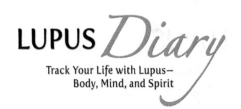 **LUPUS** *Diary*

Track Your Life with Lupus—
Body, Mind, and Spirit

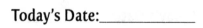 **Today's Date:**_____

Meals

Breakfast	Lunch	Dinner
_____	_____	_____
_____	_____	_____
_____	_____	_____
_____	_____	_____

Snacks	Water	Reactions to Foods
_____	_____	_____
_____	_____	_____
_____	_____	_____

Notes and Reminders

Items to remember to share with my doctor or other practitioner

_____

_____

_____

_____

_____

_____

_____

_____

_____

_____

Today's Date:_____

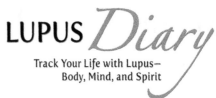

Gratitude

What am I thankful for today?

_____

_____

_____

_____

_____

_____

_____

More

More thoughts, details, feelings, aha moments about living with Lupus....

_____

_____

_____

_____

_____

_____

_____

_____

_____

_____

_____

_____

_____

_____

_____

_____

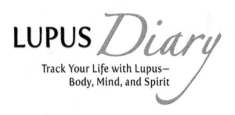
LUPUS *Diary*

Track Your Life with Lupus—
Body, Mind, and Spirit

_____
_____
_____
_____
_____
_____
_____
_____
_____
_____
_____
_____
_____
_____
_____
_____
_____

*Live life to the fullest, and
focus on the positive.*

Matt Cameron

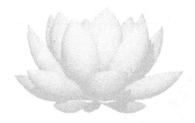

Today's Date:_____

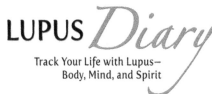

LUPUS *Diary*
Track Your Life with Lupus—
Body, Mind, and Spirit

Body

Today's Habits/Rituals to Soothe My Lupus Body:

○ Slept Well   ○ Ate a Clean Diet   ○ Got a Gentle Massage   ○ Stayed Hydrated   ○ Smiled & Laughed
○ Took a Warm Bath   ○ Moved & Stretched   ○ Breathed Fresh Air   ○ Protected Skin   ○ Was Intimate

Details and Thoughts About My Physical Symptoms Today:

_____

_____

_____

_____

Mind

Today's Habits/Rituals to Strengthen My Lupus Mind:

○ Managed Expectations   ○ Asked for & Accepted Help   ○ Focused on the Positive   ○ Forgave & Released   ○ Connected
○ Managed Time & Energy   ○ Protected Alone Time   ○ Managed Stress Response   ○ Learned About Lupus   with My Doctor

Details and Thoughts About My Emotions Today:

_____

_____

_____

_____

Spirit

Today's Habits/Rituals to Nurture My Lupus Spirit:

○ Enjoyed Sacred Space   ○ Cultivated Creativity   ○ Embraced Uncertainty   ○ Loved Myself
○ Meditated, Prayed, Visualized   ○ Made Someone Happy   ○ Worked on Finding and Living My Purpose

Details and Thoughts About My Spiritual Connection Today:

_____

_____

_____

_____

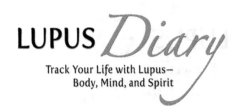

Meals

Breakfast

_____
_____
_____
_____

Lunch

_____
_____
_____
_____

Dinner

_____
_____
_____
_____

Snacks

_____
_____
_____
_____

Water

_____
_____
_____
_____

Reactions to Foods

_____
_____
_____
_____

Notes and Reminders

Items to remember to share with my doctor or other practitioner

_____
_____
_____
_____
_____
_____
_____
_____
_____
_____
_____
_____

Today's Date:_____

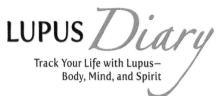

LUPUS *Diary*

Track Your Life with Lupus—
Body, Mind, and Spirit

Gratitude

What am I thankful for today?

_____

_____

_____

_____

_____

_____

_____

More

More thoughts, details, feelings, aha moments about living with Lupus....

_____

_____

_____

_____

_____

_____

_____

_____

_____

_____

_____

_____

_____

_____

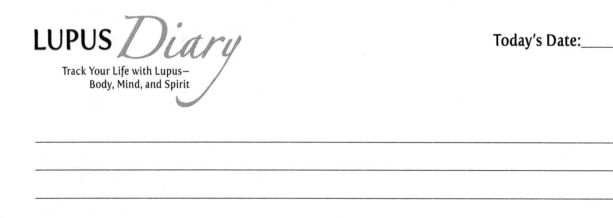

LUPUS *Diary*

Track Your Life with Lupus—
Body, Mind, and Spirit

_____
_____
_____
_____
_____
_____
_____
_____
_____
_____
_____
_____
_____
_____
_____
_____

*Since habits become power,
make them work for you,
and not against you.*

E. Stanley Jones

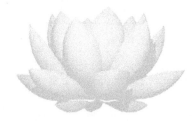

Today's Date:_____

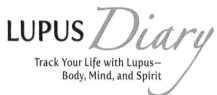

LUPUS *Diary*

Track Your Life with Lupus—
Body, Mind, and Spirit

Body

Today's Habits/Rituals to Soothe My Lupus Body:

○ Slept Well   ○ Ate a Clean Diet   ○ Got a Gentle Massage   ○ Stayed Hydrated   ○ Smiled & Laughed
○ Took a Warm Bath   ○ Moved & Stretched   ○ Breathed Fresh Air   ○ Protected Skin   ○ Was Intimate

Details and Thoughts About My Physical Symptoms Today:

_____

_____

_____

_____

Mind

Today's Habits/Rituals to Strengthen My Lupus Mind:

○ Managed Expectations   ○ Asked for & Accepted Help   ○ Focused on the Positive   ○ Forgave & Released   ○ Connected
○ Managed Time & Energy ○ Protected Alone Time   ○ Managed Stress Response ○ Learned About Lupus   with My
                                                                                                          Doctor

Details and Thoughts About My Emotions Today:

_____

_____

_____

_____

Spirit

Today's Habits/Rituals to Nurture My Lupus Spirit:

○ Enjoyed Sacred Space   ○ Cultivated Creativity   ○ Embraced Uncertainty   ○ Loved Myself
○ Meditated, Prayed, Visualized ○ Made Someone Happy   ○ Worked on Finding and Living My Purpose

Details and Thoughts About My Spiritual Connection Today:

_____

_____

_____

_____

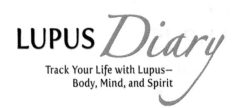

LUPUS *Diary*

Track Your Life with Lupus—
Body, Mind, and Spirit

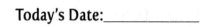

Today's Date:_____

Meals

Breakfast

_____
_____
_____
_____

Lunch

_____
_____
_____
_____

Dinner

_____
_____
_____
_____

Snacks

_____
_____
_____

Water

_____
_____
_____

Reactions to Foods

_____
_____
_____

Notes and Reminders

Items to remember to share with my doctor or other practitioner

_____
_____
_____
_____
_____
_____
_____
_____
_____
_____
_____
_____

Today's Date:_____

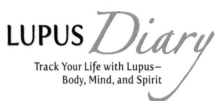

LUPUS *Diary*
Track Your Life with Lupus—
Body, Mind, and Spirit

Gratitude

What am I thankful for today?

_____
_____
_____
_____
_____
_____

More

More thoughts, details, feelings, aha moments about living with Lupus....

_____
_____
_____
_____
_____
_____
_____
_____
_____
_____
_____
_____
_____
_____
_____

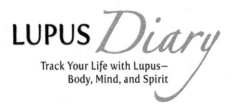

LUPUS *Diary*
Track Your Life with Lupus—
Body, Mind, and Spirit

Today's Date:_____

_____

_____

_____

_____

_____

_____

_____

_____

_____

_____

_____

_____

_____

_____

_____

_____

*You have power over your mind—
not outside events. Realize this,
and you will find strength.*

Marcus Aurelius

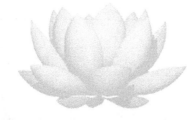

Today's Date:_____

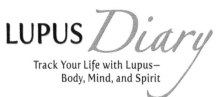

Body

Today's Habits/Rituals to Soothe My Lupus Body:

○ *Slept Well*   ○ *Ate a Clean Diet*   ○ *Got a Gentle Massage*   ○ *Stayed Hydrated*   ○ *Smiled & Laughed*

○ *Took a Warm Bath*   ○ *Moved & Stretched*   ○ *Breathed Fresh Air*   ○ *Protected Skin*   ○ *Was Intimate*

Details and Thoughts About My Physical Symptoms Today:

_____

_____

_____

_____

Mind

Today's Habits/Rituals to Strengthen My Lupus Mind:

○ *Managed Expectations*   ○ *Asked for & Accepted Help*   ○ *Focused on the Positive*   ○ *Forgave & Released*   ○ *Connected with My Doctor*

○ *Managed Time & Energy*   ○ *Protected Alone Time*   ○ *Managed Stress Response*   ○ *Learned About Lupus*

Details and Thoughts About My Emotions Today:

_____

_____

_____

_____

Spirit

Today's Habits/Rituals to Nurture My Lupus Spirit:

○ *Enjoyed Sacred Space*   ○ *Cultivated Creativity*   ○ *Embraced Uncertainty*   ○ *Loved Myself*

○ *Meditated, Prayed, Visualized* ○ *Made Someone Happy*   ○ *Worked on Finding and Living My Purpose*

Details and Thoughts About My Spiritual Connection Today:

_____

_____

_____

_____

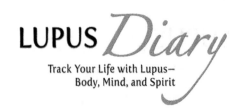

LUPUS *Diary*

Track Your Life with Lupus—
Body, Mind, and Spirit

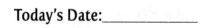

Today's Date:_____

Meals

Breakfast

_____
_____
_____
_____

Lunch

_____
_____
_____
_____

Dinner

_____
_____
_____
_____

Snacks

_____
_____
_____

Water

_____
_____
_____

Reactions to Foods

_____
_____
_____

Notes and Reminders

Items to remember to share with my doctor or other practitioner

_____

Today's Date:_____

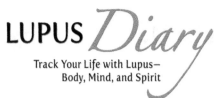

LUPUS *Diary*
Track Your Life with Lupus—
Body, Mind, and Spirit

Gratitude

What am I thankful for today?

_____

_____

_____

_____

_____

_____

_____

More

More thoughts, details, feelings, aha moments about living with Lupus....

_____

_____

_____

_____

_____

_____

_____

_____

_____

_____

_____

_____

_____

_____

_____

_____

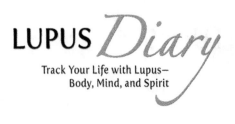
LUPUS *Diary*

Track Your Life with Lupus—
Body, Mind, and Spirit

_____

_____

_____

_____

_____

_____

_____

_____

_____

_____

_____

_____

_____

_____

_____

_____

*Have patience with everything that
remains unsolved in your heart....
Live in the questions now.*

Rainer Maria Rilke

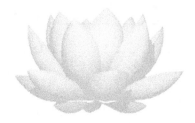

Today's Date: _____

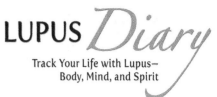

Body

Today's Habits/Rituals to Soothe My Lupus Body:

○ Slept Well   ○ Ate a Clean Diet   ○ Got a Gentle Massage   ○ Stayed Hydrated   ○ Smiled & Laughed
○ Took a Warm Bath   ○ Moved & Stretched   ○ Breathed Fresh Air   ○ Protected Skin   ○ Was Intimate

Details and Thoughts About My Physical Symptoms Today:

_____

_____

_____

_____

Mind

Today's Habits/Rituals to Strengthen My Lupus Mind:

○ Managed Expectations   ○ Asked for & Accepted Help   ○ Focused on the Positive   ○ Forgave & Released   ○ Connected with My Doctor
○ Managed Time & Energy   ○ Protected Alone Time   ○ Managed Stress Response   ○ Learned About Lupus

Details and Thoughts About My Emotions Today:

_____

_____

_____

_____

Spirit

Today's Habits/Rituals to Nurture My Lupus Spirit:

○ Enjoyed Sacred Space   ○ Cultivated Creativity   ○ Embraced Uncertainty   ○ Loved Myself
○ Meditated, Prayed, Visualized   ○ Made Someone Happy   ○ Worked on Finding and Living My Purpose

Details and Thoughts About My Spiritual Connection Today:

_____

_____

_____

_____

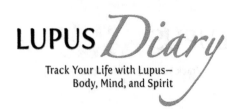

LUPUS *Diary*

Track Your Life with Lupus—
Body, Mind, and Spirit

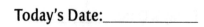

Today's Date:_____

Meals

Breakfast

_____
_____
_____
_____

Lunch

_____
_____
_____
_____

Dinner

_____
_____
_____
_____

Snacks

_____
_____
_____
_____

Water

_____
_____
_____
_____

Reactions to Foods

_____
_____
_____
_____

Notes and Reminders

Items to remember to share with my doctor or other practitioner

_____
_____
_____
_____
_____
_____
_____
_____
_____
_____
_____
_____

Today's Date:_____

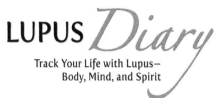

Gratitude

What am I thankful for today?

_____

_____

_____

_____

_____

_____

_____

More

More thoughts, details, feelings, aha moments about living with Lupus....

_____

_____

_____

_____

_____

_____

_____

_____

_____

_____

_____

_____

_____

_____

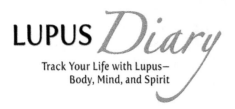

LUPUS *Diary*

Track Your Life with Lupus—
Body, Mind, and Spirit

_____
_____
_____
_____
_____
_____
_____
_____
_____
_____
_____
_____
_____
_____
_____
_____

The most authentic thing about us is our capacity to create, to overcome, to endure, to transform, to love, and to be greater than our suffering.

Ben Okri

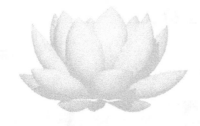

Also by Olivia Davenport

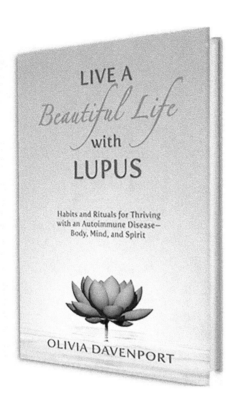

LIVE A BEAUTIFUL LIFE WITH LUPUS:
Habits and Rituals for Thriving with an Autoimmune Disease—
Body, Mind, and Spirit

ISBN: 978-0-9967498-4-4 (paperback)
ISBN: 978-0-9967498-3-1 (ebook)

Available at Bookstores Everywhere

About the Author

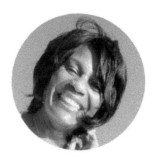

Author, blogger, and former overachiever Olivia Davenport wants to spread the news that you can live a beautiful life with Lupus. She suffered with mysterious illnesses and life-threatening episodes for over 20 years before finally getting a diagnosis of Lupus in 2012. It was then that she began a journey of research and self-discovery, to determine the habits and rituals to support her goal of not losing herself to the incurable autoimmune disease.

Lupus Diary: Tracking Your Life with Lupus—Body, Mind, and Spirit is the companion to her first book, *Live a Beautiful Life with Lupus: Habits and Rituals for Thriving with an Autoimmune Disease—Body, Mind, and Spirit*, which is available in print and Kindle e-book formats.

Olivia also maintains two websites, *www.liveabeautifullifewithlupus.com* and *www. lupusdiary.com*, where she finds joy in sharing her life, her inspirational insights, and what she's learning about Lupus.

Olivia lives in Reno, Nevada with her Hubby and their odd-eyed cat, Kitty-Witty.

Printed in the USA
CPSIA information can be obtained
at www.ICGtesting.com
LVHW010059131023
760672LV00061B/1457